Cleanse Your Body, Clear Your Mind

Cleanse Your Body, Clear Your Mind

Eliminate Environmental Toxins to Lose Weight,
Increase Energy, and Reverse Illness in
—— **30 DAYS OR LESS** ——

Jeffrey A. Morrison, M.D.

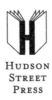

HUDSON
STREET
PRESS

HUDSON STREET PRESS
Published by Penguin Group
Penguin Group (USA) Inc., 375 Hudson Street, New York, New York 10014, U.S.A. • Penguin Group (Canada), 90 Eglinton Avenue East, Suite 700, Toronto, Ontario, Canada M4P 2Y3 (a division of Pearson Penguin Canada Inc.) • Penguin Books Ltd., 80 Strand, London WC2R 0RL, England • Penguin Ireland, 25 St. Stephen's Green, Dublin 2, Ireland (a division of Penguin Books Ltd.) • Penguin Group (Australia), 250 Camberwell Road, Camberwell, Victoria 3124, Australia (a division of Pearson Australia Group Pty. Ltd.) • Penguin Books India Pvt. Ltd., 11 Community Centre, Panchsheel Park, New Delhi – 110 017, India • Penguin Books (NZ), 67 Apollo Drive, Rosedale, North Shore 0632, New Zealand (a division of Pearson New Zealand Ltd.) • Penguin Books (South Africa) (Pty.) Ltd., 24 Sturdee Avenue, Rosebank, Johannesburg 2196, South Africa

Penguin Books Ltd., Registered Offices: 80 Strand, London WC2R 0RL, England

First published by Hudson Street Press, a member of Penguin Group (USA) Inc.

First Printing, April 2011
10   9   8   7   6   5   4   3   2   1

REGISTERED TRADEMARK—MARCA REGISTRADA
HUDSON
STREET
PRESS

LIBRARY OF CONGRESS CATALOGING-IN-PUBLICATION DATA

Morrison, Jeffrey A.
Cleanse your body, clear your mind : eliminate environmental toxins to lose weight, increase energy, and reverse illness in 30 days or less / Jeffrey A. Morrison.
p.   cm.
Includes index.
ISBN 978-1-59463-076-7 (hardback)
1. Detoxification (Health)—Popular works.   2. Nutrition—Popular works.   3. Self-care, Health—Popular works.   I. Title.
RA784.5M66 2011
613—dc22   2010046520

Printed in the United States of America
Designed by Daniel Lagin

PUBLISHER'S NOTE
Every effort has been made to ensure that the information contained in this book is complete and accurate. However, neither the publisher nor the author is engaged in rendering professional advice or services to the individual reader. The ideas, procedures, and suggestions contained in this book are not intended as a substitute for consulting with your physician. All matters regarding your health require medical supervision. Neither the author nor the publisher shall be liable or responsible for any loss or damage allegedly arising from any information or suggestion in this book.

*To my grandparents—Molly and Sam Morrison,
and Sylvia and Louis Lockett—whose love and wisdom
helped give me the confidence to explore my own
theories on health and healing.*

*To Adam Symons, my best friend from childhood,
who passed away much too soon. Our curiosity and adventures
inspired me to seek a better understanding
and appreciation of our fragile environment.*

Contents

Acknowledgments   ix

Introduction: Why Detox?   xi

Part I: Identifying Toxins   1

1. The Body Burden   3

2. The Symptoms of Toxicity   17

3. Identifying Sources of Environmental Toxins   32

4. Eliminating Toxins in Your Home   59

5. Is Your Diet Making You Sick?   80

Part II: The Effect of Toxins on Health   99

6. Good Health Begins with Clean Cells   101

7. Clear Your Mind for Better Thinking   111

8. Reduce Inflammation and Improve Immune Function   122

9. Resolving Digestion and Weight Issues   142

10. Reversing Cardiovascular Disease and Diabetes   160

11. Correcting Hormone Imbalances   173

Part III: The 30-Day Detox

Part III: The 30-Day Detox — 183

12. Get Ready to Detox — 185
13. The Meal Plan — 201

Conclusion: Day 31 and the Seven Steps
to Lasting Health — 227

Appendix I: Supporting Your Detox:
Nutritional Supplements and More — 235

Appendix II: Questions for Your Doctor
and Additional Testing Options — 255

Appendix III: Additional Resources — 261

References — 263

Index — 267

Acknowledgments

This book could not have been possible without the gracious help of many important people. I would first like to thank my parents, Marti and Jerry, for continuing to be extremely supportive of my ambitions and interests, particularly in this unique field of environmental medicine. My mom has always given me a great deal of emotional guidance, especially when I didn't know if I had the endurance to overcome my uncertainties in writing this book. My dad has always given me the practical advice and strong work ethic to finish any project with the same drive and determination that I started with.

I would also like to thank my staff at The Morrison Center: Grace, Denise, Sevgi, Jerry, Onica, Cymon, Alex, David, and Jackie—I really appreciate how all of you were able to endure my frequent schedule modifications and mood swings. Shanel, thank you for your fantastic recipe suggestions, many of which I included in this book.

I would like to thank Pam Liflander—who patiently sat with me and tape recorded, organized, and edited my thoughts into this book. My literary agents, Laura Yorke and Carol Mann, introduced me to a spectacular team at Hudson Street Press, and I'm thrilled to have worked with Caroline Sutton and Meghan Stevenson. I would also like to thank

Judy Taylor and Jennifer Ruff for introducing me to Laura and Carol, making this entire project possible.

I owe my gratitude to my good friend Jessica Tran, who absolutely wouldn't let me rest until I completed my clinical outcome studies. And finally, I would like to thank my patients, for sharing their stories, and letting me into their lives.

Introduction
Why Detox?

Many of my patients come to see me because they are suffering from medical conditions like chronic fatigue syndrome, fibromyalgia, irritable bowel syndrome, memory changes, hypertension, mercury poisoning, difficulty focusing, irritability, arthritis, high blood pressure, hormone imbalance, obesity, diabetes, anxiety, or depression. Often, their health impacts their lives to the point of debilitation. Yet within the first thirty days of following my detox program, they are usually experiencing significantly better health. You can too.

My goal is to take the science of detoxification to a new level and to teach you about the real toll of toxic exposure. By understanding the issues our lifestyle and environment pose, you will be able to successfully link your current medical conditions to specific environmental concerns, and then reverse the damage by removing harmful toxins or behaviors from your life.

We are living in a world that even our parents wouldn't easily recognize. Not only have we created considerable technological advancements, but we have also created pollution. The fact is, there is no place on earth where man-made chemicals are not detectable.

Despite our best intentions, each of us continues to ingest tiny amounts of chemicals every day, and they are making us sick. The Environmental Protection Agency (EPA) estimates that there are more than twenty thousand different types of chemicals that our bodies cannot metabolize. In fact, our bodies have become repositories for the thousands of compounds that have invaded our air, water, and food supplies:

- More than seventy-seven thousand chemicals are in active production in North America alone.
- More than ten thousand of those chemicals—in the form of solvents, emulsifiers, and preservatives—are used in food processing, packaging, wrapping, and storage.
- More than three thousand of those chemicals are added directly to our food supply.

Our bodies accumulate these toxins like autumn leaves that land in a gutter. When they overwhelm our ability to eliminate them through the skin, lungs, liver, and kidneys, they are stored in fat cells inside our body and block its ability to function correctly. That is why these chemicals are increasingly linked to failing health.

The body reacts in an attempt at self-protection by swelling up with excess water and additional fat. At the same time, the damage caused by toxins can lower metabolism, which can make us gain weight even if we are constantly dieting. They can also cause enzyme dysfunction, nutritional deficiencies, and hormonal imbalances, damage our brain chemistry, and affect our health on a cellular level. What's more, they are very possibly linked to cancer, infertility, and numerous other health problems.

I define toxins not simply as health-threatening substances but as any type of dangerous overexposure that causes dysfunction in the body. This can include chemicals, heavy metals, or poor nutrition. These toxins affect each of us differently: they can be stored in various parts of the body, at different rates, and in different combinations. This is why there is a disturbingly large variety of chronic illnesses linked to chemical exposure. While you might not be aware of the effects chemicals can have on your body, you may already be experiencing signs and symptoms linked to excess exposure, which can include:

- allergies
- difficulty concentrating
- digestive gas and bloating
- fatigue
- headaches
- irritability
- low mood
- muscle aches
- obesity
- poor memory

Yet astonishingly, conventionally trained physicians and health professionals rarely understand how our toxic environment can impact our health or know how to treat its related conditions. They are often unaware of the latest scientific findings on chemical exposure, leaving them poorly prepared to advise patients about proactive care. This leaves individuals like you in the dark, trying to figure out why their symptoms and conditions simply won't go away.

If you are experiencing any of these conditions, there is new hope. You can take control of your health with a thorough and effective whole-body detoxification program.

By doing so, you may quickly see a complete reversal of illnesses, especially of chronic ailments that have been plaguing you without relief.

By following this program for as few as ten days, you will begin to:

- Lose weight
- Restore health
- Increase energy
- Reduce brain fog
- Develop an improved sense of well-being
- Create a new healthy lifestyle with lasting results

Why Detox?

In my many years of clinical work as a board-certified family practice doctor who focuses on environmental medicine, I have found that a nutritional approach to health care is often more effective than conventional treatments. The majority of patients' problems can be significantly improved by diet modification. The most common medically related killers in the United States are heart disease, high blood pressure, and diabetes; yet if a person follows a healthy diet, it significantly lowers the risk of developing these conditions or further problems. My practice focuses on preventing and reversing degenerative and chronic diseases. I treat my patients with specific protocols, including detoxification programs that are aimed at enhancing the body's ability to naturally heal itself.

Detoxification programs have fallen in and out of favor for hundreds of years. Most of us probably associate them with their use in eliminating alcohol or drugs from a person's life. But today "detox" has come to mean giving up certain foods and behaviors with the goal of creating a healthy lifestyle modification. Through the body's own functional process of elimination, we can retrain our internal organs to become better at healing themselves. Cells will work better at producing energy and eliminating waste. Body tissue will become better able to get rid of excess toxins that have built up, with the result that internally swelling reduces and externally skin color looks better. Eventually, circulation improves, which leads to a lower risk of high blood pressure, heart disease, and diabetes as well as improved liver and kidney function.

Recently, detox diets have achieved notoriety due to celebrity endorsements and marketing suggesting quick-and-easy weight loss. You may have heard of the Master Cleanse or raw food detoxification, neither of which is practical for long-term use, and both of which can actually overwhelm the body's systems. Instead, we need a detox program that can do more, work better, and truly cleanse our bodies and restore our health. That's why I've created a totally new program that yields excellent results without having to fast, compromise our health, or deprive our taste buds or lifestyle.

Best of all, this detox is inexpensive. You'll find that you are eating out less and cooking at home more, which saves money. More important, by adopting better lifestyle choices now, your health care costs down the road can actually decrease. Preventative medicine is known to reduce the need for prescription medications and surgeries as well as lessen the likelihood of developing heart disease, diabetes, or high blood pressure. It is a short-term investment in your health that leads to long-term payoffs. Ultimately, it is the least expensive health care option available.

Why Me?

Although my training as a family practice physician was as traditional as it gets, I've always been interested in new, more organic ways to treat my patients. Back in 1999 I began practicing environmental medicine with Dr. John Sullivan. Under his guidance, I learned about the connection between pollutants and chemical sensitivities, heavy metal toxicity, and the broad range of food and environmental allergies. Dr. Sullivan and I coauthored an article about a novel approach to treating endometriosis, which was published in *Alternative and Complementary Therapies* in August 1999. We found that diet modification and detoxification is effective for women with endometriosis. Since then, I've realized that many health complaints can be resolved once the body's burden of toxicity is lowered.

I continued my training with the American Academy of Environmental Medicine, a four-part elective program that educates physicians about how to identify and treat overexposure to chemicals, heavy metals, and mold as well as sensitivities and allergies to certain foods. It is a wonderful resource to help health care providers broaden their understanding of how modern living has negatively impacted our health.

Two years later, I came to New York City to practice with famed diet guru Dr. Robert Atkins. It was an opportunity I could not pass up: he was a famous doctor, with a thriving practice, who was particularly interested in having someone on board with a concentration in environmental medicine. Atkins treated many patients in need of detoxification as well as weight loss.

Working with Dr. Atkins paved the way for me to open my own practice in 2002. I became the go-to doctor for people whose ailments conventional medicine was not able to help because I was able to find the connections between their illnesses and the toxic problems in our environment.

How This Book Works

This book will teach you exactly how different chemicals and lifestyle choices negatively affect the body. First, I will help explain the latest scientific data that links toxins to specific illnesses. I'll discuss the types of chemicals that are currently known to cause health problems, where they come from, and how they affect our health. In addition, I'll share the best strategies for limiting exposure and explain how to improve your innate ability to detoxify chemicals from your body.

You will take a simple quiz that will help you link your current symptoms with possible toxicity. Then you'll learn how you can begin an easy detox program, eliminating the toxins that have been stored within your body. This is not a "one size fits all" approach: you will be able to tailor the program to your specific needs. Then you'll learn how to stay on the program for lasting health.

The book will also provide complete information on how to make lasting dietary changes in order to provide better nutritional support for optimal body function. You'll soon understand how proper nutrition can improve the detoxification process. Then I'll share my comprehensive lists of delicious fresh foods to eat (and the ones to avoid) as well as meal plans and sample menus that will make detoxing easier than ever before. You'll learn about all the necessary supplements you may need to take to restore and support better health in the future.

I hope that you will join me for the next thirty days. You'll find that the plan is fast and yields results. Other detox programs can take up to fourteen weeks to work: you'll see positive changes to the way you look and feel in as few as ten days. Best of all, when you follow this program you'll find that it makes a true, lasting change in your entire way of life.

Part I
Identifying Toxins

All things are connected. Whatever befalls the
earth befalls the children of the earth.

—CHIEF SEATTLE OF THE SUQUAMISH
AND DUWAMISH

Chapter 1
The Body Burden

The human body deals with toxins like a barrel that is being continuously filled with water. Once the barrel is completely full, the water starts pouring over the sides. If toxic exposure is limited—i.e., before the barrel is full—we won't notice that it is causing health problems. But once the body reaches that tipping point where it can't handle another drop, its resources for detoxification become dysfunctional and illness results. When the body can no longer detoxify on its own, we put ourselves into a situation where our internal organs become exposed to toxins, which then begins to have detrimental effects.

Of the tens of thousands of chemicals we are exposed to every day, scientists estimate that we all carry at least seven hundred contaminants in our body, regardless of whether we live in a rural area, a large city, or near an industrialized zone. Some chemicals stay inside our bodies for only a short time before we naturally dispose of them through the body's own detoxification processes: digestion/elimination, breathing, and sweating. Yet continuous exposure to these chemicals leaves more than a residual trace. Worse, some chemicals cannot be automatically removed from the body and remain in our blood, fat tissue, muscles, bones, brain tissue, and other organs. All of these chemicals contribute to our "body burden": the total amount of these chemicals that are present in the human body at a given point in time.

And just as each of us is a unique and distinct individual, we each handle body burdens differently. Some of us are better than others at detoxifying the body. Whether your body is good or bad at it probably has to do with genetics. This is why toxins affect some of us more than others.

Aside from chemical exposure, we also produce toxins within our bodies during the daily process of living: through diet, digestion, and elimination, when we are combating disease or infection, and when we are dealing with stress. Some people produce additional toxins as the result of food allergies or sensitivities. These various internal and external exposures can also overburden our inherent detoxification systems, which is why we need to aid the body in order to regain full health.

The goal of an effective detox program is to lower your body burden. If you can modify your diet and eliminate exposure to the things that are causing you to be sick, then your body will have a chance to heal itself and get rid of toxins more efficiently. I believe that the easiest way to lower the body burden is by modifying the largest vehicle of exposure: the foods we eat. When toxic foods are avoided, it leaves your basic diet quite clean.

Along with better diet, you may need additional nutritional supplements that enhance your body's ability to detoxify itself. Once you've successfully limited your exposure, the body will sense that it's a good time to start using its own mechanisms to localize and eliminate new toxins quickly and efficiently. A good detox process is basically an intensive care plan to give your body an opportunity to start pulling the toxins out of their storage places and get them out of your system.

A Lesson in Biology

Let's begin by better understanding how your body detoxifies itself and where it needs help. We'll address the six major organs where detoxification takes place. This basic biology lesson shows both sides of detox: how the body works when everything is going fine and how detoxification fails when the load is too big for it to handle.

The Skin

The skin is the largest organ of the body, but very few people know that the skin is one of our most efficient detoxification organs. When the liver and kidneys, our primary sources of detoxification, aren't working at their optimal level, the skin takes over.

When the body is detoxing correctly, it excretes water and toxins via sweat. Sweat is produced in glands that are connected to millions of tiny hair follicles found in the pores of our skin. When the body becomes overheated due to infection, inflammation, or exposure to a toxin, our internal temperature rises. Sweat is one way in which we can instantly bring that temperature down to cool us. Some people also sweat under stress, but that's not related to the detoxification process. Actually, detoxification through sweat occurs primarily during sleep. Because we detoxify best when we are sleeping, poor sleep, or difficulty in falling asleep can be signs of poor detoxification capacity, or a toxic body. A body at rest is more efficient at detoxification; thus sweating from saunas is more effective for detoxifying than sweating from exercise.

Sweat carries away salt and other chemicals from our body. We know that heavy metals come out of the body through the skin during dry sauna therapy, and so do other types of chemicals that we are exposed to. In fact, almost any chemical can be excreted through the skin.

Our skin shows us how our body is functioning. When we are healthy and detoxification comes easily, the skin has a healthy color and glow and it feels soft and slightly moist to the touch. Yet when the skin does not look healthy, frequently something is not right inside. When the body is unable to detoxify, the skin will erupt with dry patches (psoriasis), red patches (eczema), bumps (hives), or rashes. Some people might notice acne or oily skin, or that their sweat becomes gritty or has a strong smell. These are all signs that the internal organs are becoming overwhelmed by some type of toxin.

The Nose and Upper Airway

The nose is the portal to our body's airway, allowing us to breathe clean, filtered, and humidified air. When you breathe in through your nose—which you should—air travels past scroll-like structures called turbinates and through your sinuses on its way to the lungs. The major function of the turbinates and sinuses is to warm and humidify the air that we breathe so it arrives in the lungs ready for oxygen to be extracted from it for use in the rest of the body. A special tissue covers the turbinates and sinuses, called mucosal epithelium, which produces mucus to protect the airway and filter the air.

The upper airway responds to the constantly changing environment. Air is cleaned and prepared so it reaches the lungs free of contaminated particles. The airway removes pollution (dirt, dust, or car exhaust), irritating agents (toxins, chemicals, smoke, etc.), allergens (pollen, ragweed, mold, etc.), and organisms (bacteria, fungus, virus, etc.) that may be carried in the air.

When the upper airway is functioning properly, you are able to breathe easily and clearly through your nose. However, when you are exposed to irritants or chemicals the lining in your nose can become worn down, which makes previously non-allergenic material like dust, pollen, and mold stimulate an allergic immune response. Once an allergy response is provoked, you'll keep getting allergy symptoms every time you come into contact with that allergenic material. In other words, every time you're exposed to dust, you'll find you have a stuffy nose, post nasal drip, and sinus congestion. Also, certain foods can worsen this type of reaction: eating dairy products can increase mucus production and create a worsening of symptoms, which is why your mom always told you not to eat dairy products when you had a cold. Symptoms from allergic reactions are very similar to those of a cold, so often it is difficult to distinguish between a cold and allergies. One of the typical signs that you have an allergy and not a cold is that along with symptoms like sneezing and coughing you also have itchy eyes or itchy ears. Also, if the "cold symptoms" are present every spring, or do not respond to cold medicines, you may be dealing with allergies and not an infection.

The Lungs

Once air is processed in the nose and upper airway, it moves toward the lungs through the trachea, which divides into two branches, or bronchi, each feeding into one lung. Within each lung, the bronchi further divide into thousands of smaller branches, forming the bronchial tree. Each branch is surrounded by rings of muscles that constrict and relax in response to various stimuli as we breathe, allowing air to flow freely. The air eventually reaches the alveoli, where the exchange takes place among the network of blood vessels that surround it: with every breath the lungs inhale air with the goal of absorbing oxygen in exchange for exhaling carbon dioxide, along with toxins.

However, airborne irritants can work their way into the lungs and over time may cause or contribute to inflammation and asthma, a condition in which the muscles surrounding the bronchi tighten, significantly reducing their size. This is referred to as an acute (sudden) asthma attack, which causes airway obstruction. Meanwhile, the mucous membrane that lines the trachea and bronchi begins to swell and produce more mucus, further obstructing the bronchi. When the airways become severely narrowed and obstructed, there is very limited airflow and greater effort is needed to get the proper amount of air into the lung. This is similar to what happens if you get a splinter in your finger. At first you may not even notice that you have a splinter, but, sure enough, if you don't do something about it, your body will start creating swelling and inflammation around the splinter, which the body identifies as a foreign intruder. This is the immune system's way of trying to get rid of the splinter on its own. The only way to stop the immune response in the finger is to pull out the splinter. However, in the lungs there could be thousands of irritating pollen molecules that can't be avoided until the end of the allergy season, triggering a continuous immune response that can get progressively worse.

The mucus clogging the bronchial tubes becomes thickened and may become infected, causing a chronic cough and shortness of breath. The lungs will begin to wheeze. The wheezing is the high-pitched sound of air pushing through the bronchi as it tries to get in or out of the lungs. Asthma symptoms can also include chest pain and rapid breathing, or hyperventilation.

A classic triad of symptoms is seen with asthma:

- cough
- shortness of breath
- wheezing

These symptoms may occur simultaneously or only one may occur at a time. When they do occur, it is a sure sign that the body is having an immune reaction, and the goal is then to identify the underlying causes of the reaction and limit or remove them so the symptoms can be prevented from occurring.

The Kidneys

The kidneys are located on either side of your lower back, just underneath the rib cage in an area called the retroperitoneum. They are responsible for regulating blood pressure, producing the active form of vitamin D, and controlling the production of red blood cells. Every day the kidneys process about two hundred quarts (190 liters) of blood and filter out nearly two quarts (1.9 liters) of extra water and waste products. These can include prescription medications, excess hormones, chemicals, heavy metals, and extra electrolytes and minerals. After that fluid is filtered in the kidneys, it drains through muscular tubes into the bladder, where urine collects and is temporarily stored until the bladder fills to capacity, which is when you get the urge to urinate. Then liquid waste passes out of the body.

Just as the skin is a way we can determine our overall health, we can see the effects of toxins in the color and odor of our urine. The healthiest urine is pale yellow in color and completely odorless. Urine can change color or smell based on what you eat or are exposed to. For example, if you eat asparagus, it might smell strong. If you take a vitamin B supplement, your urine will be bright yellow. However, when the body becomes toxic, the kidneys may become damaged or dysfunctional, and you can see that in your urine as well. This can also happen because of diabetes, high blood pressure, or heart disease or from damage caused by prescriptions or over-the-counter medications, other toxins, pesticides, or street drugs.

The symptoms of kidney dysfunction are not often obvious until there is a great deal of kidney damage. The signs can include puffiness around the eyes or fluid retention in both hands and feet that does not resolve after a good night's sleep. But if your urine consistently smells sweet, has a pinkish or brown color, and/or makes bubbles in the toilet, you should see a doctor. There are many reasons for kidney dysfunction, all of which warrant medical attention.

The Liver

The liver has the most comprehensive job of all our organs; it is truly the workhorse of the body. It is the only organ capable of regenerating itself if damaged by trauma, toxic poisoning, or surgery. It is the largest of the internal organs, occupying the entire space underneath your right rib cage. It has a filtering capacity of one quart (.9 liters) of blood every minute, and it has unique metabolic functions. The liver not only breaks down and recycles red blood cells, converting a waste product into a useful component of digestion, but also stores glucose to maintain consistent blood-sugar levels and energy. It also stores multiple vitamins and processes numerous toxins, from alcohol to car exhaust.

As blood flows through the liver, chemicals are captured in cells and undergo a three-part process of detoxification. During phase one, chemicals are activated and prepared for processing in phase two. This process creates an activated toxic intermediate, which is often more harmful to the body than the original toxin, so if this process is not handled efficiently, you can become sick. During phase two, the toxic intermediate is made water soluble and changes to a nontoxic substance, so it can be transported out of the liver safely. Transport proteins chaperone the substance out of the liver, through the gallbladder, and out of the body in the third part of the process.

Another simple way to evaluate your health is by looking at your bowel movement (BM). In medical school I was taught that we should have at least one BM per week, but after watching clients detoxify, I've come to recognize that at least one to three daily is extremely important for proper detoxification purposes. A healthy BM is brown, about the width of a sausage, and shaped like an S or a banana.

On the other hand, unhealthy BMs come in a variety of colors and shapes. If your stool is black, this can suggest upper intestinal bleeding. If it looks red, then it could be a sign of lower intestinal bleeding or hemorrhoids. If it looks green, it is a sign that your body is dumping bile rather than reabsorbing it properly. Thin BMs suggest that there is not enough fiber in the diet or that there is an imbalance of good bacteria in the digestive tract. Food particles suggest rapid intestinal transit and possibly poor absorption of nutrients. If it floats, that suggests poor fat absorption. Smelly BMs or intestinal gas and bloating are typically from bad bacteria or an imbalance of intestinal bacteria with intestinal yeast but can also be suggestive of food sensitivity or fermentation of food.

The BMs that most often suggest poor liver detoxification are rock solid. Chronic constipation is the sign of an overworked liver, while chronic diarrhea is suggestive of intestinal inflammation. If you experience either of these symptoms for an extended period of time, you should seek medical advice.

The Lymphatic System

The lymphatic system is a separate circulatory system that supports your immunity, acting like an internal sewage system. Tissues become filled with toxic debris from daily, normal bodily functions or from immune cells that have defeated invaders. Our body removes the bad stuff from our tissues and carries it through the bloodstream to be processed by the liver. This occurs through a network of conduits called the lymphatic system, which in addition to its responsibilities as a sewer also absorbs and transports fats and fatty acids as well as immune cells.

Normally, the lymphatic system works smoothly and efficiently. However, once our body has accumulated lots of chemicals, has chronic untreated infections, or has experienced trauma to the lymphatic tissue, the lymphatic system can back up. Symptoms of this include swelling of the tissue in the hands, feet, and legs that indents when pressed firmly. Also, it is thought that cellulite and fatty tumors (lipomas) are signs of poor lymphatic drainage.

Health Concerns That Influence Body Burden

By understanding how your body is intended to work, you can begin to identify if you are currently suffering from a toxic exposure. Just as chemical exposure affects body burden, your current health can also affect how well your system can detoxify. Three main areas to consider are the relationship between weight, stress, and genetic susceptibility to past exposure.

Weight Gain

There's a lot of speculation as to why people have difficulty losing weight, ranging from the foods we eat, to changes in metabolism, to current health status. I've found that there is a distinct relationship between body burden and holding on to extra weight. Often people have difficulty losing weight because their body is toxic. The relationship between weight gain and toxic exposure is particularly straightforward: the more toxins you get exposed to, the more toxins you store. When toxins overwhelm our ability to detoxify, they are stored in fat cells, specifically the type that is difficult to get rid of through dieting alone. The storage system for toxins actually works in much the same way that excess calories are stored as body fat.

Another possibility is that the body stores toxins in fluid, which is why some people have persistent fluid retention and swelling. Once the body has created these toxic fat cells or swellings, it's not so willing to release them. A toxic body may intentionally hold on to excess fat or fluid to prevent being re-exposed to the toxins as they pass out of the body. In other words, our own body is protecting us from the toxins that we've accumulated by holding on to excess weight rather than risk re-exposure. Imagine you do a big cleanup in your yard after a rainstorm and end up with a great deal more garbage than usual. You may decide to store all the trash bags in the garage until the garbage collectors come to take them away. However, what if the roads are blocked and the garbage collectors can't get to your house? The garbage piles up and becomes difficult to manage, making it increasingly difficult for you to get your car into the garage. When we can't remove toxins from our own body, they begin to pile up in the same manner, eventually affecting our health.

Interestingly, people who do not have a buffer of extra fat but are exposed to chemicals often experience worse outcomes and more toxic effects than people who might be a little overweight. Just imagine what happens to your very lean friend if he gets exposed to chemicals. Since there is not enough body fat to accept the toxins, they end up getting deposited in the site of the next highest fat content, the brain. Anecdotally, I've noticed that thin patients who visit my practice tend to be more sensitive to chemicals, fragrances, or other environmental exposures and more apt to develop difficulty concentrating and experience memory changes.

Another reason why we gain weight during times of poor detoxification has to do with how the body deals with a toxic overload. When you're overloaded with chemicals, the body transfers its energy away from burning calories and puts that energy into its detoxification response. The body literally doesn't have the energy to burn calories. But on the flip side of this, when we reduce the exposure to chemicals, our body is better able to focus on getting rid of the excess fluid it has been retaining and to start burning the fat where the toxins are stored, and thus to lose weight.

The last link between weight gain and poor detoxification is the food we choose to eat. We require food as our energy source. The more nutritious the food, the better our body will work. The more calories a person consumes, the more chance there is for the body to start storing fat. If we can select our calories from nutrient-rich foods that are free of toxins, then our body will receive the best nutrient intake and we may feel satisfied with fewer calories. Many people find they are unsatisfied from eating the highly processed standard American diet. This could easily change when you choose to eat, for example, fruits and vegetables that are locally grown using organic practices that ensure the vitamins, minerals, and nutrients in the soil are transferred to them.

However, keep in mind that weight loss does not necessarily correlate to an instantaneous decrease in toxicity. Toxins can either stay in the tissue they were in, but become more concentrated, or they can circulate around the body and be deposited someplace else. It all comes down to how well the liver and kidneys are able to process them. If the detoxification routes are closed, then toxins are not going to move out of the body. That's one of the reasons why we try to combine weight loss and detoxification in this program, so that not only will you shed pounds, you'll shed toxins.

Stress

Stress results from a complex interaction between the demands of the outside world and the body's capacity to adapt to them. Unfortunately, regardless of a person's innate mental or physical capacity, normal stressors can eventually accumulate to the point that they become overwhelming.

Stress can develop from both physical and emotional sources. This book focuses on a specific group of physical sources, including chemicals, heavy metals, and poor diet. Simply put, toxins can cause physical and emotional stress. And when the body is under any type of stress—either from toxins or other aspects of your life—it becomes distracted from one of its main goals, which is to focus on detoxification.

Signs and symptoms of chronic stress can include the following symptoms:

- anxiety
- depression
- difficulty concentrating
- fatigue
- high blood pressure
- insomnia
- irregular menstrual cycles
- irritable bowel syndrome
- low libido
- memory changes
- muscle aches
- recurrent infections
- tension headaches
- weight gain

Once you can get your internal detoxification back on track, your body will be better able to manage one of its main sources of stress and, by so doing, stress levels will naturally decrease, and you will see the improvement of many of these symptoms. By following this program, you'll be able to lighten your stress load as you decrease your body burden.

Epigenetics: Not All Bodies Are Created Equal

Epigenetics is the study of how genes, and your DNA, can change depending on environmental factors and influences. These changes can be made within your lifetime or passed down from one generation to another. The nongenetic factors that can alter DNA include the type of food you are raised on and the nutrients or toxic chemicals found in those foods. For example, when Native Americans or people of Hispanic descent continue to eat a carbohydrate-rich diet full of rice and beans, these cultural groups become more susceptible to developing type 2 diabetes, high blood pressure, and heart disease. These diseases were not typical for their ancestors, who may have eaten fewer refined carbohydrates and more animal protein and vegetables. Many doctors and researchers believe, as I do, that our lifestyle and the environment have a significant impact on expression of our genetic makeup.

Our genes are basically a library that provides information to our cells about how to perform their day-to-day functions. However, genes can also trigger unwanted cellular behavior and cancer growth. For example, the *BRCA1* or *BRCA2* genes that are linked to familial breast cancer can be stimulated by exogenous estrogenic chemicals like dioxins found in industrial waste, phthalates found in skin care products, and/or plasticizers released into microwaved food from plastic containers. Epigenetics can help to explain how one person in a family gets sick and others do not. Some people in the same family can choose to eat healthier foods or prepare their food differently, thus changing their susceptibility to disease.

Even though epigenetics is a new medical frontier, doctors have been observing differences in genetic susceptibility for a long time. One of the greatest documented reviews of differences in familial health patterns based on nutritional and environmental influences was undertaken in the early 1900s by retired dentist Weston Price. He traveled the world with his wife to study the dental health of people living in indigenous cultures. He assumed that individuals who had no exposure to modern dentistry would have terrible dentition and cavities, and would be in desperate need of braces. However, what he found was the exact opposite. In fact, he managed to take photographs of groups of twins across the world, demonstrating that the twin who was raised entirely in indigenous cultures, without modern dentistry or exposure to refined foods, had almost perfect teeth, with no need for braces or fillings, while the siblings who were raised in modern cities and ate a diet of modern processed food had many cavities and needed braces because their teeth had developed poorly.

Now that you understand how detoxification works inside your body, we can begin to address your unique body burden and determine how it is affecting your health. Then you'll have all the information you need to start this program and to individualize it to get the best results.

Chapter 2
The Symptoms of Toxicity

Our health is fragile. We can wake up in the morning and feel great, or completely out of sorts, or somewhere in between. Symptoms of illness can pass quickly or become chronic. Sometimes we know exactly what is causing us to feel bad: a virus, a bacterial infection, or a diagnosis confirmed by your doctor through medical testing. Yet at other times, we experience signs and symptoms of illness that have no apparent connection to our current health status or see a group of symptoms that are seemingly unrelated. These unexplained or surprise conditions are usually the ones that bring people into my office.

While your symptoms and conditions may be caused by genetics, they can also be caused, or even exacerbated, by our toxic world. And to make things more confusing, toxins can have different effects on different people, depending on the amount, timing, duration, and pattern of exposure. I view illness as the result of many factors interacting with one another.

Each toxin can affect the body on the cellular level, which eventually leads to illness and disease. While single low-level toxic exposures generally don't cause one immediate symptom or constellation of symptoms, a single large exposure or multiple low-level exposures over time can cause cellular dysfunction. When a toxin enters our cells, they respond by trying to neutralize it with antioxidants, and then remove it from the cell to be passed out of the body through our innate detoxification process. Over time these toxins can build up, which stops the cells from functioning properly. When this happens, cells can't produce energy the way that they're supposed to and are unable to heal themselves or keep other toxins out. Most importantly, they are not able to communicate properly with the other cells in the body. This breakdown on the cellular level is why illness and organ dysfunction occurs. We'll go into this in much more detail in chapter 6. But for now it's important to see how easily your symptoms may be linked to toxicity.

Adaptation: How a Toxic Environment Can Seem Normal

Humans are a very adaptable species, so much so that our bodies continually adapt to our environment. Whether we live in Iceland or on the equator or anywhere in between, the human body is exactly the same. The differences occur in the way we choose to live our lives: the clothes we wear or the amount of time we spend outdoors.

Just as we can adapt to where we live, our bodies can adapt to different types of environmental exposures. After stepping outside on a bright sunny day, our eyes adapt to the sunlight after only a few moments. If we make a living working with our hands, it won't take long for the skin to become calloused to protect against irritation. When I was growing up, my grandmother would take my brother and me to the local pastry shop for a treat. I loved the smell of the fresh baked goods. But after a few minutes, the smell was gone. The smell hadn't actually disappeared—I had just adapted to it.

While adaptation can be useful, it becomes dangerous when chemical exposures are involved. Because adaptation can happen quickly, we sometimes miss the warning signs of a toxic threat. For example, when the body adapts to the smells of new carpeting or a moldy bathroom without reacting, you might feel that you are in a safe environment. Or if you don't realize that your digestion is off every time you eat a certain type of food, like dairy products, you will continue to eat that food. However, over time, as you spend more time in the moldy bathroom or eating dairy products, these toxic exposures are building up. Eventually, your body will develop new or aggravated symptoms that are difficult to link to toxicity. But with proper testing, you can easily see the connection.

Adaptation is just one example of why working with a doctor familiar with environmental medicine is so critical to good health. These doctors can help you track down the original cause of your symptoms and help you make good decisions about modifications that need to be made to the way you live.

The Spreading Phenomenon: Symptoms Multiply

If you are exposed to a particular chemical, it can initially cause a reaction or illness in one part of the body. For example, if you are exposed to cigarette smoke, you might start coughing. But if the exposure is large or ongoing, the number of symptoms can increase as the cigarette smoke affects other parts of the body. Regardless of whether you are the smoker or breathing secondhand smoke, you may develop asthma, sinus symptoms, and, if you are continuously exposed, cancer.

The good news is that once you eliminate the exposure, you'll find that your symptoms may go away. What's interesting is that the initial symptom will likely be the last one you will get rid of. In this same example, your sinuses will clear before your lungs, so your cough may linger long after your stuffy nose is gone.

The Switch Phenomenon: Seemingly Separate Symptoms Can Be Related

Because the body is so adaptable, symptoms of toxic exposure can change over time. This makes tracing the effects of chemical exposure highly difficult. And if a doctor is treating just your symptoms, they may go away but be replaced with another symptom or disease elsewhere in the body.

For example, if you have been told that you have asthma and are being treated with steroids, your symptoms may improve. But if you don't explore the underlying reason why your asthma flared up to begin with, you might end up with another set of symptoms that are completely unrelated, like recurrent sinus or bladder infections, even if the asthma is under control. The same toxin is affecting your body but manifesting with a different set of symptoms.

Once you identify and remove the toxin, however, your total health should improve.

Biochemical Individuality: Why "Standard" Protocols Don't Work for Everyone

Just as each of us is unique, we each have our own unique ability to detoxify or manage our body burden. That's why not every person with fillings gets mercury toxicity, not everybody who works at a gas station develops chemical sensitivity, and not everyone who has allergies gets swollen eyes in the springtime. And this is why each of us must be treated as a unique individual by our health care practitioner and not just be given the standard treatment—usually prescription medication—to reverse high blood pressure, high cholesterol, or allergies.

If I've learned anything over the course of my career, it's that individuals respond to different treatments, and all of them are worth considering. In my practice, I see patients who have seen no improvement with traditional medications respond well to acupuncture, homeopathy, or simple lifestyle modifications. This is what makes the practice of medicine an art; it is the pursuit, identification, and elimination of the cause of symptoms that, when accomplished, leaves both patient and health care provider satisfied.

Symptoms and Your Body Burden

Symptoms may at first appear insidiously, almost imperceptibly. Often by the time you recognize that you are not quite yourself, you are already experiencing a range of symptoms that can be hard to group together. For example, you may be experiencing extreme fatigue, muscle aches, joint aches, memory changes, weight gain, low mood, and digestive problems. These symptoms may be grouped together by your health care provider so that a label can be given to create a diagnosis. The labels that might be used in conventional medicine could include chronic fatigue syndrome, fibromyalgia syndrome, or irritable bowel syndrome, all of which are nothing more than names for constellations of symptoms.

A toxic environment can make some people's immune system dysfunctional, which can create allergies, asthma, and chronic infections. Or toxins can affect another organ system and cause high blood pressure, difficulty concentrating, or even menstrual irregularity. If your symptoms are recurrent or chronic, or if you've had symptoms and you've tried to treat them in other ways and they haven't gone away, the problem could be that you are sensitive to something in your environment or have accumulated too many toxins in your body.

While it's very difficult to link a specific illness to one toxin or another, there are studies that provide a handful of clear connections. Research has confirmed that overexposure to heavy metals and mercury increases the susceptibility to autoimmune disease. Exposure to the chemical bisphenol A (BPA) may be linked to hormone imbalances. Individuals with high levels of lead in their systems may be more susceptible to high blood pressure and heart disease.

Regardless of whether you are experiencing one symptom or twenty, any symptom can represent a real health concern. The problem with conventional medicine is that it will treat symptoms without necessarily finding the underlying cause of the problem. Sometimes treating the symptoms alone works: you can effectively take an antihistamine medication that controls your allergies, for example, or you may be prescribed a powerful antacid for your digestive complaints. However, if your symptoms do not go away after weeks of treatment, then it may be important for you and your doctor to look deeper and decipher the underlying cause of your illness.

My job is to help you make that connection: to see whether the symptoms you are experiencing are linked to toxins and sensitivities. If they are, you can begin the detox and see if you feel better. The first step is to figure out what symptoms you may be experiencing.

Connect the Dots: The Detox Questionnaire

The detox questionnaire will review a large range of symptoms and conditions, and then rate your level of overall toxicity based on the answers you provide, ranging from low to moderate to elevated. Once you take the questionnaire, you can better determine which areas of the body have been most affected. This will help you monitor certain symptoms during your detox.

Review the list of symptoms and conditions. Rate each one on a scale of 0 to 4 using the following scale:

0 Never experience the symptom

1 Infrequently experience the symptom (less than once a month) and the effect is mild

2 Occasionally experience the symptom (at least once a month) and the effect is modest

3 Regularly experience the symptom (at least once a week) and the effect is moderate

4 Constantly experience the symptom (every day) and the effect is severe

At the end of each section, add up your points to determine the category score. At the end of the test, add all of your points together to determine your overall score. Please take the questionnaire before you start the program, and then repeat it after thirty days to see how much your symptoms improve.

GROUP 1: NEUROLOGICAL FUNCTION					
Energy/Activity					
Apathy, lethargy	0	1	2	3	4
Fatigue, sluggishness	0	1	2	3	4
Hyperactivity	0	1	2	3	4
Restlessness	0	1	2	3	4
Insomnia	0	1	2	3	4
Mind					
Confusion, poor comprehension	0	1	2	3	4
Difficulty making decisions	0	1	2	3	4
Learning disabilities	0	1	2	3	4
Poor concentration	0	1	2	3	4
Poor memory	0	1	2	3	4
Poor physical coordination	0	1	2	3	4
Slurred speech	0	1	2	3	4
Stuttering or stammering	0	1	2	3	4

Emotions					
Anxiety, fear, nervousness	0	1	2	3	4
Depression	0	1	2	3	4
Mood swings	0	1	2	3	4
Neurological Function Total:					

GROUP 2: IMMUNE FUNCTION

Head					
Dizziness	0	1	2	3	4
Faintness	0	1	2	3	4
Headaches	0	1	2	3	4
Eyes					
Bags or dark circles under the eyes	0	1	2	3	4
Blurred or tunnel vision	0	1	2	3	4
Swollen, reddened, or sticky eyelids	0	1	2	3	4
Watery or itchy eyes	0	1	2	3	4
Ears					
Drainage from ear	0	1	2	3	4
Earaches, ear infections	0	1	2	3	4
Itchy ears	0	1	2	3	4
Nose					
Excessive mucus	0	1	2	3	4

Hay fever	0 1 2 3 4
Sinus problems	0 1 2 3 4
Sneezing attacks	0 1 2 3 4
Stuffy nose	0 1 2 3 4
Mouth/Throat	
Canker sores	0 1 2 3 4
Chronic coughing	0 1 2 3 4
Gagging, frequent need to clear throat	0 1 2 3 4
Sore throat, hoarseness, loss of voice	0 1 2 3 4
Swollen or discolored tongue, gums, lips	0 1 2 3 4
Skin	
Acne	0 1 2 3 4
Excessive sweating	0 1 2 3 4
Flushing	0 1 2 3 4
Hair loss	0 1 2 3 4
Hives, rashes, dry skin	0 1 2 3 4
Lungs	
Asthma	0 1 2 3 4
Bronchitis	0 1 2 3 4
Chest congestion	0 1 2 3 4
Difficulty breathing	0 1 2 3 4
Shortness of breath	0 1 2 3 4

Joints/Muscle					
Arthritis	0	1	2	3	4
Feeling of weakness or tiredness	0	1	2	3	4
Pain or aches in joints	0	1	2	3	4
Pain or aches in muscles	0	1	2	3	4
Stiffness or limitation of movement	0	1	2	3	4
Immune Function Total:					

GROUP 3: WEIGHT/DIGESTION FUNCTION

Weight					
Binge eating/drinking	0	1	2	3	4
Compulsive eating	0	1	2	3	4
Craving certain foods	0	1	2	3	4
Excessive weight	0	1	2	3	4
Underweight	0	1	2	3	4
Water retention	0	1	2	3	4
Digestive Tract					
Belching, passing gas	0	1	2	3	4
Bloating	0	1	2	3	4
Constipation	0	1	2	3	4
Diarrhea	0	1	2	3	4
Heartburn	0	1	2	3	4

Intestinal/stomach pain	0 1 2 3 4
Nausea, vomiting	0 1 2 3 4

Weight/Digestion Function Total:

GROUP 4: CARDIOVASCULAR AND METABOLIC FUNCTION

Chest pain	0 1 2 3 4
Frequent illness	0 1 2 3 4
Frequent or urgent urination	0 1 2 3 4
Irregular or skipped heartbeat	0 1 2 3 4
Rapid or pounding heartbeat	0 1 2 3 4
Numbness or tingling in hands and feet	0 1 2 3 4

Cardiovascular and Metabolic Function Total:

GROUP 5: HORMONE IMBALANCES

Women

Genital itch or discharge	0 1 2 3 4
Hot flashes, night sweats	0 1 2 3 4
Loss of libido	0 1 2 3 4
Painful menstrual cycle	0 1 2 3 4
Premenstrual syndrome (PMS)	0 1 2 3 4
Short or long menstrual cycle	0 1 2 3 4
Early onset of menstruation	0 1 2 3 4

Early onset of menopause	0	1	2	3	4
Fertility issues	0	1	2	3	4
Men					
Difficulty starting or stopping urination	0	1	2	3	4
Difficulty getting or maintaining erection	0	1	2	3	4
Loss of libido	0	1	2	3	4
Fertility issues	0	1	2	3	4
Hormone Imbalances Total:					

Total Score (add all five section scores together): _____

Individualized program recommendations based on your total score:

0–14 points: low toxicity; take the 10-day seasonal detox

15–49 points: take the 30-day detox plus maintenance supplements

50 or higher: start with the 30-day detox; this score suggests major health issues that need to be addressed

Many of the symptoms and conditions that are highlighted in this questionnaire can be resolved by detoxification. Part 2 of this book addresses these same groups of health concerns, with separate chapters devoted to each. You can address the areas of your health that scored highest by beginning with the corresponding chapter and making the necessary modifications to your eating plan. There are also symptom-specific supplements you can take during the 30-day program and additional detoxification therapies that address these individual concerns, which can be found in Appendix I and II.

Getting Started on the Program

You can begin the plan at any time. Don't wait for a Monday or a Sunday or the Friday after Christmas. Start taking care of your health now.

Over the next thirty days of following the plan, you will begin to feel significantly better. Statistically, my patients feel about 60 percent better in the first thirty days, which is tremendously high considering that you may have been feeling poorly for three months, six months, a year, or quite possibly your whole life. And from the outcomes that I've collected with my own patients, you can expect to lose as much as nine pounds or more over the next thirty days.

For some people, the change to better health is very rapid. For others, with more advanced illnesses, the healing process may take longer. Your results will depend on how advanced the disease process is and how well you are able to heal yourself. Generally, people believe that if you're younger, you heal better. But that's not always the case.

I suggest that you take the detox questionnaire again after the first thirty days, and then consider whether you want to continue.

If your total score does not drop at least 50 percent and is above 14, that's a sign to stick with the program as is and work with your health care provider to determine if there are other underlying causes for your symptoms that might be identified through blood work. (See appendix 2 for questions you should ask your doctor and a list of diagnostic tests divided by the symptom categories.) If your total score drops by more than 50 percent and/or is less than 15, then you can begin the second phase of the program and switch to a seasonal detox four times a year.

If your total score is under 15, you can still benefit from a full 30-day detox. However, you can also start with a 10-day version of the same plan. This score shows that you are generally well, and the 10-day plan is a great option for anybody who is interested in maintaining optimal health.

You can start the 10-day plan at any time, but if you live in a part of the country that experiences four full seasons, you may reap the best results if you start at the beginning of the spring. That is the time of year when the body is highly prepared for healing itself. In the spring our bodies want to rejuvenate after surviving the winter. Also, if you are affected by allergies a detox at that time of the year is extremely effective, and may even decrease your allergy symptoms.

While there's never been a great deal of research on this concept, I believe that a spring cleansing is part of optimizing good health. During the winter our bodies produce certain hormones to try to help us handle the stress of the colder weather. Those hormones include cortisol. A short-term cortisol increase is helpful because it improves white blood cell production, which positively affects our immune system. But when cortisol is chronically high, as it frequently is during the course of a long winter, then it makes us gain can weight and can worsen our immune system function.

A drastic example of creating too much cortisol occurs when a person takes prednisone for a long period of time. Initially, this medication, which is a synthetic form of cortisol, can make you feel quite energetic. But then if you're on it for weeks, you start feeling quite irritable, jittery, or even fatigued. Then you may start to retain fluid and gain weight. In addition, your appetite increases. These are some of the same symptoms many of us have during the winter, as we naturally increase our own cortisol production.

In the spring, when the weather starts getting warmer, our internal thermostat changes and so do many of our body functions. We don't have to try to create more heat in our body, which gives it a chance to rest. And when our body is resting, that's when it goes into a healing phase. When the body is at rest, it detoxes better—the liver works better and the kidneys work better. We may find that we have less fluid retention and less abdominal bloating in the spring.

The parasympathetic nervous system is the system that takes over control when our body is resting. During the spring, the parasympathetic nervous system is able to function better, which means that we're able to digest better, we're able to heal our tissue better, and we're able to repair our skin better. And we want to take advantage of this opportunity by giving our body the nutrients that are necessary to heal itself during this time. With the help of the detox diet, we basically eliminate the foods that might interfere with the healing process and focus on foods that are nutrient dense, with lots of antioxidants, vitamins, and minerals: the best nutrition for the body's needs.

With a spring cleansing, you can get the most out of the detoxification. However, spring is not the only preferred time. Any change of season is a good moment to start. As the seasons change, different foods become available, and our body naturally benefits from eating them. Eating the seasonal foods helps our metabolism and nervous systems adapt to the seasonal change more readily.

The Next Step: Identifying the Cause of Your Symptoms

The symptoms of toxicity are ubiquitous and can relate to many different things, so how do we know what is really causing them? Ultimately, we must find the underlying causes of disease. And luckily our body, when given the right circumstances, can heal itself.

The next few chapters will educate you more about the various toxins. Once you understand how possible exposures might affect your health, and can begin to identify their sources, you'll be ready to make the most of your detox.

Chapter 3
Identifying Sources of Environmental Toxins

The first goal of a good detox is to eliminate the toxins causing your symptoms. To do that, it's important to understand, and be able to identify, the different ways in which you may be getting exposed. It's not easy to avoid all chemicals because they are ubiquitous, and often we are exposed to them in ways that are completely out of our control. Chemicals exist in our water, air, and food, and as you'll learn in the next chapter, also in our homes. However, once you figure out which toxins are making you sick, the fix is easy. By limiting your exposure to harmful environmental substances and completing a thorough detoxification, you can begin your healing process.

When I'm not treating patients, I spend lots of time lecturing around the country, helping other doctors to understand and identify toxin exposures so they can help their patients feel better. Every year my audience grows, which is one way that I know that my message is being heard. I know I can't stop the spread of toxicity on a global scale, but I can educate. If other doctors incorporate the underlying themes of environmental medicine into their practices, they may see, as I do, that treating patients this way yields terrific and lasting results.

Even if your doctor does not practice environmental medicine, you can learn from these same tenets. You can put your own life under the magnifying glass to see how your symptoms are linked to specific exposures. Then you can begin getting rid of the things in your life that are making you sick. It might be as simple as modifying your diet or changing household cleaners and not microwaving your food in plastic containers. You may need to detoxify your house as well as your body, and knowing how to make the best consumer choices is an easy way to feel well.

You might also need to make some lifestyle changes. Your drinking water may not be as clean as you thought, the fish you eat may not be the healthiest choice, or you may need to move your daily run through city streets to a different location. Your decisions about what changes will benefit you the most will be based on what you learn in this chapter.

Government agencies like the EPA, individual researchers, and physicians are trying to understand how a variety of individual pollutants affect our health. Most testing is conducted through animal studies or by monitoring the outcomes of individuals who have been accidentally exposed to high levels of pollutants. However, it is important to recognize that the effects of multiple toxins, accumulated over time, is completely unknown and unstudied. We do not definitively know how different types of pollutants and toxins interact in the body. A major concern is that exposure to and accumulation of combinations of toxins may have magnified implications for our health, far more than we can glean from lab studies.

At the same time, it's important to keep pollution and toxins in perspective. Please don't be alarmed by what you are about to read. It can be overwhelming, and even a little frightening, to discover that the sources of toxin exposure are so widespread and commonplace. The most important thing is for you to recognize the names of these pollutants and where you are likely to come in contact with them, so you can learn strategies for avoiding them and choosing better options, and then incorporate those strategies into your daily life.

Water Contamination

Hopefully, crystal clear drinking water pours from your kitchen sink. But even if it looks good, and tastes good, that water may not be so good for you. Even the "cleanest" drinking water can contain chemicals, particulate matter, and heavy metals. According to a 2009 article published in the *New York Times*, over 20 percent of the nation's water treatment systems have violated key provisions of the Safe Drinking Water Act in the past five years. The violations include illegal concentrations of chemicals like arsenic or radioactive substances like uranium as well as dangerous bacteria often found in sewage. An article by the Associated Press stated that over the last decade drinking water at thousands of schools across the country has been found to contain unsafe levels of lead, pesticides, and dozens of other toxins. Scientific research indicates that the incidence of certain types of cancer—such as breast and prostate—has risen over the past thirty years and that this rise may be connected to toxins like those found in drinking water.

Water in its purest form is odorless, colorless, and tasteless. In New York City, where I live, there are days when the water in my apartment building has an indescribable odor as it comes out of the faucets or the showerhead. It's literally so toxic smelling that I almost have to step away and wait for the smell to pass. This is particularly disturbing because New York's drinking water is highly rated. If you start noticing that your water smells, keep in mind that it's not supposed to and that the likely culprit is either a contaminant or a so-called treatment.

Water pollution affects the water we use every day, as well as rivers, streams, and oceans, which eventually affect our food supply. The damage is so pervasive because there are so many ways that water can become polluted, including the following:

- Municipal: sewage seepage from homes
- Agricultural: waste from livestock and toxic runoff of pesticides, herbicides, or fertilizers

- Industrial: waste from paper mills, chemical manufacturing, petroleum companies, and steel manufacturing

Pollutants and toxins enter our water in a number of ways. They can be directly discharged into it from a point of contamination. They can also enter rivers and streams as runoff from eroded soil or seep into the water table from farms. And they can be spread through the air and return to our sources of drinking water in the form of acid rain.

BEWARE OF BOTTLED WATERS

Toxic water can be found in municipally treated tap water, well water, and some bottled waters. In fact, many bottled waters start as municipally treated tap water, which is then put into bottles with a few added minerals or flavors to enhance the taste. Or the water may be passed through a charcoal filtering system and then bottled in the same fashion. The ideal bottled water, in my opinion, comes from a mountain spring whose water is naturally filtered by the mountain and kept pure in aquifers deep in the ground before being pumped out through a well and into glass bottles for consumption. Two national brands that currently do this are the Saratoga Spring Water Company (www.saratogaspringwater.com) in the Adirondack foothills of New York State and Mountain Valley Spring Water in Arkansas (www.mountainvalleyspring.com).

Toxins Commonly Found in Drinking Water

There are four main types of contaminants that can be found in drinking water regardless of where you live or whether your drinking water comes from a well, a municipal system, or a designer label:

- **Organic chemicals:** Despite their name, organic chemicals are man made and contain the element carbon. They include three major chemical classes: trihalomethanes (THMs), pesticides, and volatile organic compounds (VOCs), which are described in detail below. Organic chemicals can be produced by industry (VOCs and pesticides) or can be a by-product of water treatment (THMs). Organic chemicals slowly accumulate in the body, collecting in fat tissue and in the brain, and cause cellular and organ damage.

- **Inorganic chemicals:** These include toxic heavy metals like lead and mercury. They are minerals or elements found in nature that do not contain carbon and have an adverse effect on human health. When these contaminants are consumed, they can accumulate in the body over time, causing cellular dysfunction and organ damage. Throughout this chapter you'll learn more about these heavy metals.

- **Microbial pathogens (parasites and coliforms):** These pollutants enter the water system by way of untreated water from septic tanks, farm runoff, or boats that dump sewage. Even though the pathogens are microscopic, they can be quite damaging to the body through the spread of intestinal and skin diseases. Symptoms of exposure, after eating foods washed in contaminated water or drinking contaminated water (think Montezuma's revenge), might include upset stomach, loose bowel movements, or constipation. Topical exposure can cause contact dermatitis, skin infections, or even complicated internal infections if contaminated water gets into the body through an open wound.

- **Radioactive elements (including uranium and radon):** Radioactive minerals and gasses can dissolve in well water or water that is downstream from uranium mines. Drinking water that contains radioactive elements can, over time, increase the risk of developing cancer. However, you are unlikely to know if you are getting exposed to radiation until it is too late. Radiation has no smell or taste, and the only way to determine its presence is to proactively test for it. If radon levels are high in your water, then they are likely to be high in the air of your home as well, increasing your risk of developing lung cancer. For more information on radon visit the EPA's Web site (http://www.epa.gov/radon/index.html).

Trihalomethanes (THMs)

The chemicals in this class form when the chlorine and/or bromine used to disinfect drinking water mixes with human or animal feces from sewage. Although chlorine and bromine are meant to work as antibiotics or disinfectants, to kill off bacteria and parasites, not only do they help to create this toxic compound, but when we ingest water treated with them, they continue to act like an antibiotic that disinfects our digestive tract. Thus we are unknowingly taking excess antibiotics, even when we aren't sick. Trihalomethanes are also considered carcinogenic in high concentrations.

A second problem associated with water treatment is the excess chlorine left in drinking water. This will have a particularly pungent smell reminiscent of your local swimming pool.

The good news is that chlorine can be released from tap water by allowing it to sit before drinking. In my office I performed a slightly accidental science experiment with two of my Siamese fighting fish, or bettas. I placed one betta into a bowl filled with New York City tap water that had sat out overnight and the other into a bowl filled with water that came right out of the tap. Sure enough, the one that went into the fresh tap water died right away, while the other survived, probably because the chlorine was released from the water (and into the air) overnight.

You can also remove chlorine and other toxins from your water with a charcoal filter. The ones that work best are those that allow the water to travel over the most charcoal for the longest period of time: the permanent filter systems installed under a sink. The second best option is a countertop filter like the Pur Advantage pitcher. I like this one because it filters out both chemicals and parasites. I don't recommend the filter that screws onto a faucet, because it does not allow the water coming through enough contact with the charcoal to make a significant difference.

CHLORINE ALTERNATIVES FOR SWIMMING POOLS

A 2004 study presented at the American College of Sports Medicine showed an incidence rate of over 60 percent for exercise-induced bronchoconstriction (also known as exercise-induced asthma) after several minutes of swimming in water chlorinated at a concentration commonly found in home drinking water and public pools: one part per million.

If swimming is your primary form of exercise, choose your pool wisely. Some private pools, and even some public ones, are switching from chlorine and using less-toxic options, including saltwater pools, carbon filters, ozone treatments, and ultraviolet technologies.

Volatile Organic Compounds (VOCs)

These chemicals contain carbon and are found in solvents, degreasers, and gasoline additives like methyl tert-butyl ether (MTBE). Other VOCs include benzene, trichloroethylene, and styrene (used to make Styrofoam cups). Nitrates found in fertilizers, sewage, and animal wastes are all considered to be VOCs. The EPA has reported that the presence of VOCs in drinking water is a concern for human health because they can cause cancer, organ dysfunction, poor coordination, and brain dysfunction, and can adversely affect fertility.

MTBE is among a group of chemicals known as oxygenates that are added to gasoline because they raise its oxygen content, thereby acting as an antiknock agent. MTBE is not classified as a human carcinogen; however, it makes other chemicals more toxic. Possible chronic health effects include cancer, central nervous system disorders, liver and kidney damage, reproductive disorders, and birth defects.

Despite the fact that MTBE is being phased out of gasoline, it is still problematic because it breaks apart very slowly and can remain in the water supply for decades. It can be found in drinking water when fuel storage tanks leak near water supply wells. It negatively affects the taste and odor of drinking water even at very low concentrations. For example, the San Francisco Bay Regional Water Quality Control Board has indicated that MTBE is one of the groundwater pollutants of most widespread concern in that region.

VOCs AND THE SUPERFUND

The Environmental Protection Agency (EPA) offers a wealth of information about pollutants and what the government is doing about them. The agency's mission is to protect human health and to safeguard the natural environment, including our air, land, and water supply. The EPA accomplishes this mission by developing and enforcing regulations, giving grants, studying environmental issues, and providing educational resources about the environment.

A special EPA program called the Superfund was established in 1980 to locate, investigate, and clean up uncontrolled or abandoned hazardous waste sites throughout the United States. Today there are thousands of active waste sites and hundreds that are considered to be a top priority. VOCs and many other toxins are found in these sites and in the water surrounding them.

If you believe that your water—or your health—has been affected by VOCs or any other chemical toxin, you can enter your zip code or region into the Superfund list simply by visiting the Web site (www.epa.gov/superfund/sites/).

Organic Water Pollutants Are Linked to Toxic Food Exposure

All this dirty water eventually ends up on our dinner plates. Back in 1993 barely 10 percent of U.S. lake acres and only 2.5 percent of river miles were considered to be contaminated; now almost 35 percent of U.S. lake acres and over 20 percent of river miles have a pollution problem. The National Listing of Fish Advisories database includes three thousand toxic water sites in forty-eight states, the District of Columbia, American Samoa, and three Native American reservations. The number of water bodies under advisory represents fourteen million lake acres, eight hundred thousand river miles, 65 percent of the nation's contiguous coastal waters, 92 percent of the Atlantic coast, 100 percent of the

Gulf coast, and 100 percent of the Great Lakes. Think about this the next time you are offered freshly caught fish or if you enjoy fishing with your family.

Although currently advisories have been issued in the United States for thirty-six different pollutants, the three types of organic bioaccumulative contaminants most commonly found in the food supply are polychlorinated biphenyls (PCBs), dioxins and/or furans, and plasticizers.

Polychlorinated Biphenyls (PCBs)

Among the biggest food contaminants today are PCBs, a family of man-made chemicals that were used as lubricants and coolants in many commercial and electrical products because of their high resistance to heat. The EPA banned the use of PCBs in the United States in late 1970s, but almost forty years later they can still be detected in our food supply. PCBs remain at the bottom of rivers and streams. Plankton feed on them, and fish feed on plankton. The chemicals accumulate in the fat of the fish and other animals we eat, and then remain in the human body's fat stores. Studies of women and their children show a link between elevated levels of PCBs in the mothers' bodies and the birth weight, short-term memory, and learning disabilities of the child. Another study of older adults who frequently ate fish containing PCBs suggests that higher exposures are associated with decreased memory and ability to learn. Other studies have suggested links between PCB exposure and effects on the human reproductive system, including changes in sperm quality and menstrual cycles, as well as an association with cancer.

Dioxins and Furans

These closely related families of chemicals are unwanted by-products of manufacturing. They are released in smoke or ash from municipal waste incineration, wood fires, and household trash burning, as well as in the exhaust of motor vehicles. Dioxins and furans are some of the most toxic man-made chemicals that persist in the environment and accumulate in the fat of fish and other animals, which is why they are considered to be a food contaminant.

In adults dioxins and furans have been associated with severe acne, skin rashes, liver damage, weakened immune system, chemical sensitivity, allergies, obesity, fatigue, and certain cancers and developmental disorders. In children exposure can cause impaired neurological development resulting in abnormal behavior, decreased motor skills, decreased short-term memory, and decreased intelligence. They can also lower the immune system function in children, leading to allergies and chronic infections.

Unfortunately, it is not easy to determine if you have accumulated these chemicals because they are stored in fat tissue; however, the Metametrix PCBs Profile listed in appendix 2 may be a helpful tool to assess your level of exposure. You can minimize your exposure by eating either 100 percent grass-fed beef or the leanest cuts of conventional meat, selecting either organic dairy or low- or nonfat conventional dairy products, and abiding by local and state fishing advisories.

Plasticizers: Phthalates and Bisphenol A (BPA)

These chemicals are used in the manufacturing of plastic products: they allow plastics to become soft and pliable. Phthalates can leach into food when you heat or microwave in plastic wrap or plastic containers, including plastic baby bottles. They also can leach into water from plastic bottles that become hot from sun exposure. If you ever drank water from a plastic bottle that tasted funny or smelled like plastic, you were recognizing the phthalates in your water.

Plastic shopping bags are also a problem because they are photodegradable: over time and with exposure to the sun they break down into smaller, more toxic petropolymers. These microscopic particles enter the food chain as they contaminate our soil and waterways.

BPA is considered to be an endocrine disruptor or xenoestrogen, a class of compounds that when found in the body can suppress male hormones and mimic female hormones by binding with estrogen receptors. In adults endocrine disruptors are thought to increase the risk of hormone-related cancers such as those of the breasts, ovaries, and prostate. In children researches believe they may cause the early onset of puberty in girls and possibly feminization of male fetuses during gestation. While the research is still in preliminary stages, I believe that it is probably best for pregnant mothers to avoid plastics altogether.

If you do use plastics, the safer choices are those marked for recycling as numbers 1 (PET or PETE), 2 (HDPE), 4 (LDPE), and 5 (PP). Avoid plastics with the recycling codes 3 (plastic wrap), 6 (Styrofoam), and 7 (others, except new specially labeled bioplastics). Chapter 4 covers the problems with plastics in greater detail.

Mercury: An Inorganic Water Pollutant

One of the unexpected by-products of the use of fossil fuels is the release of the heavy metal mercury. When coal is burned for fuel, mercury is released into the atmosphere and then returns to earth with rain. Over time ponds, lakes, and oceans become polluted with small amounts of this heavy metal, which settles at the bottom, where the cycle of its accumulation into the food chain begins. Like many of the other toxins we've discussed, mercury accumulates in plankton and algae, which are eaten by fish, which in turn store the mercury in their fat tissue. Eventually, we consume the fish and expose ourselves to relatively large amounts of methylmercury.

Symptoms of mercury poisoning are highly varied and often nonspecific. Many times there is no correlation between the degree of mercury toxicity and the symptoms experienced. If you have any of the following symptoms and no specific cause for them has been found, get yourself tested for mercury poisoning.

- anemia
- bone marrow disorders
- depression
- difficulty concentrating
- disturbances of taste or smell
- dry mouth
- excessive perspiration
- excitability
- facial pallor (white)
- fatigue
- fearfulness
- increased salivation
- increased risk of autoimmune diseases
- indecisiveness
- insomnia
- irritability
- kidney malfunction
- loss of appetite
- melancholy
- memory changes
- nasal irritation
- nerve pain (neuralgia)
- nosebleeds
- numbness in extremities (paresthesia)
- poor digestion
- poor gait (ataxia)
- restlessness
- shyness
- speech defects
- tongue tremor
- tremor in fingers arms and legs
- tremor of eyelids
- uncontrolled blushing
- weakness

Mercury Levels and Fish

Because mercury is so pervasive, state governments carefully monitor fish and the contaminants in it. Right now the entire Atlantic coast and Gulf of Mexico are under a fish advisory. So if you're eating fish and live on the East Coast, it's very likely that you are becoming exposed to mercury and other heavy metals.

The good news is that there are plenty of fish that have low levels of mercury. Some very good online resources are available to help you determine the amount of mercury you will ingest from a given serving of fish, including Got Mercury? (www.gotmercury.org) and the FDA Web site (www.cfsan.fda.gov). The following chart offers the basic rules for choosing some of the least toxic fish.

AVOID	NOT MORE THAN ONCE PER MONTH	LOWEST IN MERCURY
Shark	Mahimahi	Catfish (farmed)
Swordfish	Blue mussel	Blue crab (mid-Atlantic)
King mackerel	Eastern oyster	Croaker
Tilefish	Cod	Fish sticks
Tuna (including canned)	Pollock	Flounder (summer)
Sea bass	Great Lakes salmon	Haddock
Gulf Coast oysters	Gulf Coast blue crab	Trout (farmed)
Marlin	Channel catfish (wild)	Salmon (wild Pacific)
Halibut	Lake whitefish	Shrimp (but keep in mind
Pike		that shrimp fishing and
White croaker		farming causes serious
Walleye		environmental damage)
Largemouth bass		

BENEFITS OF FISH DON'T NECESSARILY OUTWEIGH THE RISKS OF TOXICITY

For the past decade or so, doctors the world over have been touting the health benefits of eating fish, which is low in calories and often full of important nutrients, including omega-3 fatty acids. So it's no surprise to me that there is confusion over the issue of fish toxicity. Do the benefits of eating fish outweigh the risks?

To my mind the answer is no. In my opinion there is no acceptable limit for mercury in the blood. Once mercury is in your body, it is very difficult to get rid of without proper detoxification, which includes avoidance. This is especially true for pregnant women, because mercury can be transferred to the fetus through the placenta. When this happens, the fetus concentrates it and will not be able to eliminate it.

While the American Heart Association supports the findings that fish is beneficial to lower triglycerides and decrease the risk of heart disease, I believe that fish oil supplements that are molecularly distilled and tested for chemical toxins and heavy metals are a better resource. Choose fish oils that are tested for these toxins at parts per billion, not parts per million, and are high in the omega-3 DHA, because this helps to improve brain development and function.

Other Sources of Food Toxicity

Other sources of food contamination fall into a handful of categories that can be easily avoided.

Packaging

Aluminum or tin cans are lined with a plastic created with phthalates that leaches into food. Plastic containers used to package food and even those labeled as "microwave safe" are also potential sources of chemicals that can leach into food. A 2009 Canadian study found the estrogen-mimicking chemical bisphenol A in the vast majority of canned beverages: sixty-nine out of seventy-two individual cans tested contained residues. The highest levels of BPA were found in the linings of caffeine-loaded energy drinks, but high levels were also detected in ginger ale, diet cola, root beer, and citrus-flavored soda.

A better choice: buy fresh or frozen foods or ones that are stored and preserved in glass containers. Also, consider avoiding canned beverages: if you need caffeine, drink freshly brewed green tea.

Hormones Added to the Food Supply

Protein sources such as milk and other dairy products, beef, pork, lamb, veal, chicken, and eggs may all contain high levels of hormones. Growth hormone and genetically engineered hormones like rBGH have been systematically given to animals to stimulate faster growth and increase milk production. They are thought to possibly interfere with your health by affecting your own hormone balance. Symptoms could include early onset of puberty as well as acne, premenstrual syndrome, polycystic ovary, and obesity.

A better choice: buy certified organic meats, poultry, and dairy products that are hormone free.

Preservatives

Chemicals are often used to keep foods fresh for long periods of time. These preservatives are made from potent antioxidants that slow down the metabolic process that naturally continues even after fresh foods are packaged. The preservatives act as agents that prevent mold and bacteria from growing because they inhibit their cellular function. However, when we eat foods with preservatives they can directly interfere with our cellular function as well, by slowing down our metabolism and artificially preserving our internal systems as they preserved the food we eat.

A better choice: buy fresh and, ideally, locally grown organic proteins, fruits, vegetables, and grains that are free of preservatives.

BACTERIA IN FOODS CAN BE TOXIC

Robert Kenner's movie *Food, Inc.* did a very good job of showing how cows raised eating grain instead of their natural diet of grass develop toxic bacteria in their digestive tract that can be transferred to undercooked beef, pork, or poultry. When these animals are fed grass, which is their natural diet, the levels of toxic bacteria are almost undetectable. Look for the words "100 percent grass fed" on packages of meat and poultry.

Genetically Modified Foods

Genetically modified organisms (GMOs) have been scientifically enhanced or engineered by the insertion or deletion of genetic material in the organism's original genome. The inserted genes may come from bacteria, viruses, insects, animals, or even humans. Many fresh fruits and vegetables are now deliberately altered to make them more resistant to a certain pest or pesticide or to increase their shelf life. However, because this science is so new many of these foods have not been studied to determine their safety.

GMOs have been in the food supply since 1996 and are now present in the vast majority of processed foods in the United States. Although banned by food manufacturers in Europe, the FDA does not require any safety evaluations of GMOs, nor does it require food manufacturers to label these foods. This means that often you have no idea if your food has been altered. For more information and help in identifying whether the foods you buy contain GMOs visit the Institute for Responsible Technology Web site (www.responsibletechnology.org).

Choosing Organic Is Important

"Organic" has become an official food-labeling term that denotes food products grown or raised under the authority of the Organic Foods Production Act. Organic food production meets strict government and self-policing standards that are thought to reduce health risks because they avoid hormones, antibiotics, and GMOs. From a philosophical point of view, organic farming respects water resources and builds healthy soil: its tenets are based on the minimal use of pesticides or nonfarm-produced fertilizers and on agricultural management practices that restore, maintain, and enhance ecological harmony. Organic agriculture practices cannot ensure that products are completely free of contaminants; however, they do include methods to minimize pollution from air, soil, and water.

The benefits of eating organic are enormous. Because organically grown plants do not have the artificial protection offered by chemicals, they begin to produce higher quantities of natural antioxidants to fight off invading organisms on their own. We in turn benefit from these higher levels of antioxidants when we eat the organic produce. Studies of the nutrient content of organic foods vary due to differences in organic farming operations. However, as my friend Walter Crinnion, ND, showed in his 2010 article in *Alternative Medicine Review*, organic foods do provide significantly greater levels of vitamin C, iron, magnesium, and phosphorus than nonorganic varieties of the same foods.

Supporting local farmers is valuable for both your health and your community. When you buy from local growers, your money goes to small family farms instead of to agribusiness. The USDA reports that in 1997 half of U.S. farm production came from only 2 percent of farms. This means that nonorganic and chemically ridden farming practices produce the highest yield of crops. Organic agriculture can be a lifeline for small local farms because it offers a competitive advantage for fair prices. For more information on choosing organic, visit the Organic Trade Association Web site (www.ota.com).

Local and organic produce, poultry, meats, fish, and eggs can be found in season at farmers' markets and often even in the largest of supermarkets. Another way to support local farmers is to participate in community supported agriculture (CSA) and get your produce direct from the farms. By doing so, you financially support local organic growers and literally reap their harvest. Local CSAs deliver fresh fruits and vegetables in season to their members throughout the year. For more information about joining a CSA, visit the Local Harvest Web site (www.localharvest.org).

Air Contamination

The quality of the air we breathe is constantly affected by environmental factors like wind and rain. It is also affected by air contaminants. The EPA monitors air quality trends and reports its findings on its Web site (www.epa.gov/airtrends/index.html). Aside from this resource, or a large-scale notice of chemical contamination from an unforeseen disaster (such as 9/11 or an industrial meltdown), it isn't easy to determine if your air is affected by contaminants, regardless of whether you live in the city, the suburbs, or elsewhere. Many times contaminants have no odor or color. Common symptoms might include respiratory irritation, coughing, a stuffy nose, or watery eyes. In other instances, as is the case with carbon monoxide poisoning, there is no detectable symptom until it is too late.

The three major sources of air contamination are car and truck emissions, indoor air and industrial air pollution, and commercial emissions. The EPA, under the Clean Air Act, established air quality standards to protect our health and the environment from six common air pollutants. The good news is that over the last thirty years emissions of these six toxins have dropped by 54 percent.

Carbon Monoxide (CO)

Carbon monoxide (CO) is a colorless gas produced by vehicle exhaust, gas stoves, and kerosene space heaters. It can cause harmful health effects by reducing oxygen delivery to all body organs and is especially detrimental to the heart and nervous systems, which have high oxygen needs. Prolonged exposure can cause permanent disability or death.

Solution: use CO monitors in the home to ensure no leaks.

Ground-Level Ozone

Ground-level ozone is a gas found in smog, which is created by a chemical reaction that occurs in auto and industrial exhaust in the presence of heat and sunlight. Ozone is very irritating to the lungs, so it will worsen asthma, bronchitis, and emphysema. It also can damage vegetation, reducing crop production.

Solution: check current air quality information on ozone pollution at the EPA's AirNow Web site (http://www.airnow.gov) and limit outdoor activities when the readings are high.

Lead

Lead is a naturally occurring heavy metal. Before lead was removed from gasoline in the late 1980s, the major sources of lead emissions were car and truck exhaust. Lead is still emitted from waste incinerators and lead-acid battery manufacturers. The most common sources of lead poisoning are deteriorating lead-based paint (in homes built before 1978), lead-contaminated dust, and lead-contaminated soil. Health concerns for children include reduced IQ and hyperactivity. In adults lead can cause high blood pressure, memory changes, and muscle and joint pain.

Solution: a professional should remove lead paint; read more about lead-avoidance solutions in chapter 4.

Nitrogen Dioxide (NO$_2$)

Nitrogen dioxide occurs in a group of highly reactive gasses emitted from cars, trucks, buses, and power plants, which are involved in the formation of ground-level ozone gas and fine-particle pollution. NO$_2$ causes irritation in the respiratory track leading to asthma, bronchitis, and emphysema.

Solution: check the air quality in your area on the EPA's AirNow Web site (http://www.airnow.gov) and limit outdoor activities when the readings are high.

Particulate Matter

Particulate matter is a complex mixture of extremely small particles and liquid droplets made up of nitrates, sulfates, VOCs, heavy metals, and soil or dust particles. The size of the particles is directly linked to their potential for causing health problems. Smaller particles, less than ten micrometers in diameter, cause the greatest health problems including irritated airway, cough, difficulty breathing, decreased lung function, asthma, bronchitis, and increased risk of heart disease. Many of the same symptoms are experienced by people exposed to construction or demolition debris, including the firemen, policemen, and other individuals who were part of the rescue efforts after the 9/11 World Trade Center bombings.

Solution: avoid walking or playing near active construction sites.

Sulfur Dioxide

Sulfur dioxide is found in a group of highly reactive gasses formed by fossil-fuel combustion from vehicles, power plants, and industrial facilities. Exposure to sulfur dioxide irritates the respiratory tract and leads to an increased incidence of asthma, bronchitis, and emphysema.

Solution: close car windows and use the recycled air setting when traveling behind trucks and buses until local municipalities and businesses replace old diesel buses and trucks with cleaner alternatives.

Hazardous Air Pollutants (HAPs)

Hazardous air pollutants (HAPs) are substances known to cause, or are suspected of causing, serious health problems such as reproductive issues, birth defects, and cancer as well as having other adverse environmental effects. The EPA is working with state and local governments to reduce the release of 188 HAPs. Examples of these air pollutants include benzene, perchloroethylene (emitted from some dry cleaning facilities), trichloroethylene (TCE), methylene chloride (a solvent and paint stripper), asbestos, toluene, and the heavy metals cadmium and mercury. In 2009 the EPA released the results of its 2002 national-scale assessment of air toxin emissions, which found that there are 81 different air toxins that may be linked to cancer. The most common offenders are listed below.

Trichloroethylene (TCE)

A VOC that looks like water, vaporizes quickly, and has a sweet odor like chloroform. It was once used as a medical anesthetic but is now mainly used in metal degreasing; as a raw material to make other chemicals; as a cleaner in electronics, iron, and steel manufacturing; to sterilize medical equipment; and for general solvent purposes such as removing paints and adhesives. It has also been used as a low-temperature refrigerant and a grain fumigant, and is still often used in dry cleaning.

TCE is of particular concern because it enters your body when you breathe its vapors and can also be absorbed through your skin, especially with prolonged skin contact. Its main effect is on the central nervous system, causing headaches, nausea, dizziness, clumsiness, drowsiness, and other effects like those of being drunk. It can also damage the facial nerves and cause skin rashes, and heavy exposure can cause liver and kidney malfunction.

Cadmium

A naturally occurring heavy metal found in soil and water. It becomes vaporized during the processes of hazardous-waste incineration, cigarette smoking, wildfires, smelting of lead and copper, and from burning coal. It's used mainly for industrial operations and consumer products such as paints, plastics, and nickel-cadmium batteries. Cadmium can be found in fruits, vegetables, cereals, and tobacco because it's used in fertilizers as an insecticide. Cadmium can also be found in fish and shellfish in some waters. Cadmium accumulates mainly in the kidneys and with continued exposure can adversely affect those organs as well as bone and blood.

Benzene

A colorless liquid with a sweet odor. It evaporates into the air very quickly and dissolves slightly in water. It's highly flammable and is formed from both natural processes and human activities. Outdoor air contains low levels of benzene from tobacco smoke, automobile service stations, exhaust from motor vehicles, and industrial emissions. Vapors from products that contain benzene—such as glues, paints, furniture wax, and detergents—can also be a source of exposure. Air around hazardous-waste sites will contain high levels of benzene.

Breathing high levels of benzene can cause drowsiness, dizziness, rapid heart rate, headache, tremors, confusion, and even unconsciousness. Eating or drinking foods containing high levels of benzene can cause vomiting, irritation of the stomach, dizziness, sleepiness, convulsions, rapid heart rate, and death. The major effect of benzene is from long-term exposure and affects the blood. Benzene has harmful effects on bone marrow and can decrease the red blood cell count, leading to anemia, as well as the white blood cell count, increasing one's chances of infection.

Pesticides Affect Water, Food, and Air

Insecticides and pesticides include a broad range of products that are used in and outside the home, and on large scale in the environment. They can include fungicides that kill mold, herbicides that limit plant growth, disinfectants, and detergents as well as chemicals that kill bugs and rodents through fumigation or direct contact. They are sprayed in the air and eventually enter the water supply as runoff from farms and municipalities and homes. Pesticides also tend to accumulate in the soil and in the beds of streams, rivers, and lakes, from which they work their way into the food chain. They remain on the plants we eat and on the grain fed to the animals we eat (cows, chickens, pigs, etc.) and are ingested by the algae that are eaten by the fish we eat.

Because pesticides are fat soluble, they get stored in the fatty tissue of the animals we eat as well as in our own body fat. When these pesticides enter the body, they get stored not only around the midsection but also everywhere we have fat tissue, including our brain. This may be the reason why pesticides are associated with Parkinson's disease, as shown in a 2009 article published in *Environmental Health Perspectives.*

The scientific consensus is that pesticides stored in human fat tissue do not affect the health of other organs. However, these same pesticides may likely affect our ability to burn fat, which may be one of the reasons that some people just can't lose weight no matter how hard they try. I believe that the body is trying to protect us from re-exposure to the pesticides by keeping them stored in a relatively safe location: our fat cells. And when body fat is reduced through weight loss, these same pesticides are released into the body, which may be why some people become sick when they lose weight quickly.

In a 2006 study conducted at Université Laval in Canada, researchers found that obese patients who lost weight either through a dietary intervention or by gastroplasty (bariatric surgery) had increased levels of circulating organochlorine and pesticide compounds in their body. The amount of organochlorine and pesticide compounds correlated with the participants' ages and not their body mass (calculated as BMI). For morbidly obese individuals, the weight loss at one year after surgery yielded a 388 percent increase in total circulating pesticide concentrations. This means that the older and more overweight individuals had the largest amounts of pesticide accumulation.

Pesticide use has increased fiftyfold since 1950. Two and a half million tons of industrial pesticides are now used each year. If you live in an area near where pesticides are applied for farming or pest control, or in a city where the watershed is located near areas of pesticide application, they may be found in your drinking water or in your food.

There is growing consensus in the scientific community that small doses of pesticides can adversely affect people, especially during vulnerable periods of fetal development and childhood when exposures can have long-lasting effects. Other health concerns include links to allergies, asthma, heart disease, fatigue, frequent infections, high blood pressure, learning difficulties, and mood disorders. Pesticides have been found to cause cancer in laboratory animals. They can affect the kidneys, thyroid, and reproductive systems, and they can be transferred to growing fetuses from the placenta and to infants from breast milk.

To help minimize exposure to pesticides whenever possible, the Environmental Working Group (EWG) has created a list of foods to choose when organic options are not available. By using this list, you can lower your pesticide exposure by almost 90 percent. Eating from among the twelve most contaminated fruits and vegetables will expose you to roughly fourteen pesticides per day. Eating from among the fifteen least contaminated will expose you to fewer than two pesticides per day.

While washing and rinsing fresh produce may reduce levels of some pesticides, it does not eliminate them. Peeling also reduces exposures, but valuable nutrients are often found in the peels. Again, organic options offer the lowest levels of toxic chemical exposure.

AVOID THE DIRTY DOZEN	CHOOSE FROM THE CLEAN FIFTEEN
Peaches	Onions
Apples	Avocados
Bell peppers	Sweet corn (frozen)
Celery	Pineapple
Nectarines	Mangos
Strawberries	Sweet peas (frozen)
Cherries	Asparagus
Blueberries	Kiwi
Grapes	Watermelon
Kale	Cabbage
Spinach	Cantaloupe
Potatoes	Eggplant
	Grapefruit
	Sweet potatoes
	Honeydew melon

Types of Pesticides

Organophosphates

The most widely used insecticides. Examples include chlorpyrifos and Malathion. These chemicals are toxic to insects and mammals because of their ability to inactivate the enzyme acetylcholinesterase (AChE). Exposure in humans can cause overstimulation of nerve endings and organs, leading to headaches, excess secretion of bodily fluids, muscle twitches, nausea, diarrhea, respiratory depression, seizures, and even death. One helpful diagnostic sign is pupil constriction.

Carbamate Pesticides

Widely used in homes, gardens, and agriculture. Examples include carbaryl and carbofuran. Like organophosphates, they also inhibit the AChE enzyme and exposure therefore shares similar acute and chronic symptoms.

Organochlorine Insecticides

Commonly used in the past, they have been banned or limited in the United States due to their health effects and persistence in the environment. Examples include DDT, heptachlor, mirex, lindane, and chlordane. They are very persistent in the environment and continue to be found in fruits, vegetables, grains, meat, dairy, and fish as well as in drinking water.

Lindane is still used in the product Kwell, which is used to topically treat human lice. Lindane has a 9 percent skin-absorption rate, and children are the most likely to get symptoms from its use, including headaches, numbness and tingling in the hands and feet, increased sense of pain, dizziness, nausea, hyperexcitability, and convulsions. I recommend that instead you use a lice comb along with an alternative therapy that you and your health care provider agree upon. Lice have become resistant to many topical treatments, so oral treatments like Bactrim and ivermectin or topical prescription-strength permethrin may be better options.

Biological Pesticides

Developed as synthetic versions of naturally occurring pesticides. The pyrethroid pesticides, for example, are synthetic versions of pyrethrin, which is naturally produced in chrysanthemum flowers. Pyrethroids tend to have low toxic potential; however, commercial products may contain other toxic agents or insecticides as part of the preparation, and cases of potential overexposure should be assessed as general insecticide poisonings.

Diethyltoluamide (DEET)

A widely used insect repellent made to be applied to skin or fabrics. It is generally considered safe when used as directed on the bottle. However, DEET is so efficiently absorbed through the skin that I recommend applying it only to clothing. Symptoms of adverse effects include dermatitis, headache, irritability, loss of coordination, and low blood pressure.

Better options: natural bug repellents include citrus, catnip, neem oil, boric acid (which should not be ingested), and pyrethrin.

Fluoride

Found in toothpaste and many municipal drinking water supplies. Fluoride was once widely used to control crawling insects in homes, barns, and warehouses. The only current use is for wood treatment and toothpaste. It is highly toxic to all plant and animal life. Fluoride may help prevent cavities because it is toxic to mouth bacteria.

One sign of overexposure to fluoride is dental fluorosis: the white spots or deposits found on some people's teeth. Symptoms of fluoride overdose include thirst, abdominal pain, vomiting, diarrhea, gastric ulcerations, and, at worst, cardiac arrhythmia and shock. For these reasons I am reluctant to recommend adding fluoride to drinking water, even at low doses. Most people don't realize that the fluoride in toothpaste is actually a pesticide that kills the bacteria in their mouths. Now that you know, you can make an informed decision about whether to use toothpaste with fluoride. No matter what, don't swallow it.

Here is a summary of simple suggestions to detox your environment:

- Know your water source and learn about your local water quality at http://water.epa.gov/drink/index.cfm.
- Test well water regularly for bacteria and other toxins.
- Select spring water from a glass bottle when it is available.
- Filter your water with a countertop filter, like the Pur Advantage, or an undersink filter.
- Select lean protein sources to minimize exposure to PCBs, dioxins, furans, and heavy metals.
- Avoid using plastics for storing or cooking food.
- Choose organic foods when possible and select from the low-pesticide list if you can't find an organic option.
- Avoid genetically modified foods.
- Choose low-toxicity pesticides.
- Become active in your community to help find solutions to limit environmental pollution.

Chapter 4
Eliminating Toxins in Your Home

While it's nearly impossible to affect the majority of environmental toxins found in our air, water, and food supply, it's easy to control what we bring into our homes. Unfortunately, many of our homes are just as polluted as the outdoors. Yet by recognizing the potential problems and making lifestyle changes that address them, you can create a safe, nontoxic haven in your home.

Indoor Air Pollutants

Believe it or not, indoor air can be even more polluted than outdoor air, even in the largest industrialized cities. This is very important to recognize because we spend as much as 90 percent of our time indoors. Additionally, the people who are the most susceptible to symptoms caused by indoor pollutants—the young, elderly, and chronically ill—are the ones most likely to spend the majority of their time inside.

Indoor air is dangerous for two primary reasons: pollutants and poor ventilation. Indoor air pollution can come from home heating and cooling systems, tobacco and cigarette smoke, building material outgassing, asbestos, mold from water damage, furniture made from processed woods, household cleaners, personal care products, and air fresheners, as well as from the outdoor sources that we discussed in the previous chapter, which can become trapped indoors. Many times the air is not significantly affected by any one of these sources, but when multiple sources are added together, their individual affects can be multiplied and we can become sick.

Ventilation is an issue because new houses are built to be literally airtight, in compliance with building codes aimed at reducing the costs of heating and cooling. While we're saving money, air pollutants multiply in our poorly ventilated homes like garbage in a wastebasket.

One way to improve indoor air quality without opening the windows and letting new toxins in is by using an air purifier that can remove pollutants like pollen, dust, chemicals, and bacteria. There are many different types on the market, each with useful characteristics.

- **High-efficiency particulate air (HEPA) purifiers:** These use a fine cloth to filter and remove 99 percent of particles. The filter needs to be changed regularly and is not effective for removing gases, odors, or chemical fumes.
- **Ozone air purifiers:** These release ozone into the air to remove chemical fumes, odors, and bacteria. They are not effective for removing particles or allergens from the air, and they are not safe to run while you are in the room because ozone gas can be toxic. If you use this type of purifier, turn it off about two hours before reentering the room.
- **Carbon air purifiers:** These use activated carbon as an air filter. The carbon is able to remove odors and capture smaller particles than HEPA filters, but the carbon needs to be replaced regularly, which can be messy.
- **Ionic air purifiers:** These work by negatively charging air particles, which then attract positively charged pollutants. When the two combine, dust is created. An unwanted side effect reported with

ionizers is that they can produce ozone, so they are best turned off when people or pets are in the room.

- **Other air-purifying features** can include an ultraviolet light to kill airborne bacteria, and some air purifiers come with a combination of functions to enhance their air-cleaning ability.

The air purifiers I like best, and that I use and recommend to my patients, are made by the E. L. Foust Company (www.foustco.com). It has been in the business of making air purifiers since 1974 and its designs are created for people with environmental illnesses, allergies, or asthma.

Household Chemicals

Detergents, cleaning solvents, and indoor fragrances sound like good ideas because marketers have worked long and hard to get you interested in buying them. But the bottom line is that many are toxic and can affect your health. Besides being loaded with chemicals, many household cleaners are labeled as "antibacterial," which is just a fancy term for describing the active ingredient: pesticides.

Some scientists suggest that the overuse of cleaning agents, antibiotics, and antibacterial disinfectants to practically sterilize homes has significantly added to the number of childhood asthma and allergies cases. This is referred to as the "hygiene hypothesis."

The following ten simple tips can protect you and your family from adding to your body burden when you clean your home:

1. Dilute cleaning supplies with water, either as directed on the label or until you are happy with the results.
2. Clean with windows and doors open so you don't trap air pollution inside.
3. Use gloves: cleansers and solvents can harm or penetrate skin.

4. Never mix bleach with ammonia, vinegar, or other acids: these combinations can produce deadly gases.

5. Avoid pine and citrus oil cleaners: they may smell pleasant, but these cleaners can react with ozone in the air, particularly on smoggy days, to produce cancer-causing formaldehyde.

6. Skip acidic toilet bowl and drain cleaners: use a simple paste made out of water and baking soda and when necessary use a mechanical snake to unclog the drain.

7. Wipe down showers after each use to prevent mold and mildew growth.

8. Forget air fresheners: they only disguise odors while pumping toxic chemicals into the air.

9. Sweep and use a vacuum with a HEPA filter frequently to remove dust, which often harbors household toxins.

10. Dust with a soft or microfiber cloth and don't use toxic dusting sprays.

Natural cleaning options:

- **Baking soda:** Absorbs odors and chemicals and can be used as a mild abrasive. It can remove stains from the bathtub or toilet and remove grime from a dirty oven.
- **Borax:** A mineral compound (sodium borate) that is a disinfectant, deodorizer, mold inhibitor, and mild abrasive.
- **White vinegar:** Cuts grease, deodorizes, and dissolves sticky buildup and mineral deposits.
- **Lemon juice:** Cuts grease, dissolves sticky buildup, and has a bleaching effect.
- **Vegetable-based dish soaps:** Use a vegetable based soap that is made out of olive oil, such as castile soap.

Homemade Home-Cleaning Options

PRODUCT	HOMEMADE OPTIONS
Air freshener	1. Boil cinnamon and cloves and let the steam circulate 2. Put ½ cup of borax in the bottom of garbage pails 3. Place a box of baking soda in the refrigerator to absorb bad smells
All-purpose cleaner	Mix 1 tsp. borax, 2 tbs. vinegar or lemon juice, 5 drops essential oil of lavender, and 2 cups hot water
Tub and tile scouring powder	Mix 1 cup baking soda and ¼ cup borax, sprinkle on area, and scrub with warm water
Floor cleaner	Vinyl floors: use a mixture of ½ cup vinegar, ¼ cup borax, and 1 gallon hot water Wood floors: use a vegetable soap like castile soap or Murphy Oil Soap
Glass cleaner	Mix ⅛ cup white vinegar to 1 cup water and spray on with bottle
Furniture and floor polish	Use 2 parts olive oil, 1 part white vinegar, and essential oil for scent; another option is to use mineral oil with a few drops of lemon juice for each pint
Mold and mildew cleaner	Mix 1 tsp. borax, 3 tbs. white vinegar, and 2 cups hot water, spray on surface and scrub off mold; to inhibit mold growth spray a few more times but don't wipe off

AVOID TEFLON NONSTICK SURFACES

Teflon-coated nonstick pans can release small chemical toxins into the air when the pans are well heated, contributing to indoor air pollution. Better choices include Pyrex, cooking-grade stainless steel, or old-fashioned cast-iron cookware.

Personal Care Products

Antibacterial products are pesticides, and to my mind (and the American Medical Association's) they are overkill for general household use. If you are healthy, there's no need to use potentially toxic antibacterial products. Wash your hands with glycerine soap and water.

The problem is that antibacterial soaps contain triclosan and parabens. These chemicals are added to personal care products as antibacterial agents and to keep mold and fungi from growing in the packaging. However, both of these chemical classes are considered endocrine disruptors: compounds that suppress male hormones and mimic female hormones by binding with estrogen receptors. In adults endocrine disruptors are thought to increase the risk of hormone-related cancers like breast, ovarian, and prostate cancers. In children researchers believe that they may cause early onset of puberty in girls and may even cause feminization of male fetuses during gestation. Products that may contain parabens include cosmetics, lotions, soaps, shampoos, fragrances, moisturizers, shaving gels, and toothpaste.

And that's not all. Your medicine cabinet is full of seemingly innocuous products that could be creating symptoms and affecting your health: Antiaging creams and lotions contain lactic, glycolic, and alpha hydroxyl acids as well as BHA. Hair dyes can pollute your home with ammonia, peroxide, p-phenylenediamine, and diamino benzene. Nail polish and removers can contain phthalates (plasticizers) or formaldehyde. Deodorants and other "fragrance" products also contain phthalates.

Just because the label says "gentle," "natural," or "dermatologist tested" doesn't mean a product is safe. With no required safety testing, personal product companies can use almost any chemical they want, regardless of risks. So always read the label before you bring a product home. The first step is to understand how to read the ingredients listed on labels.

Reading Product Labels

Every personal care product must list its ingredients on its label, but the chemical names are often confusing, especially if you don't know what you are looking for. Just like FDA food labels, personal care product labels list ingredients starting with those with the highest concentration and continuing to those with the lowest. Avoid products that have the following potentially hazardous ingredients:

- PEG and anything ending with "-eth"
- benzoic acid
- BHA
- BHT
- DMDM hydantoin
- fragrance and dyes
- imidazolidinyl urea
- methylchloroisothiazolinone or methylisothiazolinone
- parfum
- sodium lauryl (laureth) sulfate
- triclosan and triclocarban
- anything ending in "paraben," such as propylparaben or methyl paraben

Look for skin products with 100 percent natural ingredients, like Tata Harper Skincare (www.tatasnaturalalchemy.com) or Farmaesthetics (www.farmaesthetics.com). Another valuable resource is the Environmental Working Group's cosmetic safety database, Skin Deep (www.cosmeticsdatabase.com). Visit it to check your personal care products for toxic ingredients.

Fire Retardants

Chemical fire retardants are commonly found in consumer products. Some of the most toxic are brominated fire retardants (BFRs), which include polybrominated diphenyl ethers (PBDEs). Exposure to even minute doses of PBDEs at critical points in development can damage reproductive systems and cause deficits in motor skills, learning, memory, and hearing as well as changes in behavior.

PBDEs are found in everyday items, including polyurethane foam products (like couches and upholstered chairs, mattresses and pads, futons, pillows, children's car seats and carpet padding), electronic equipment, lighting, wiring, building materials, textiles, furniture, and industrial paints. These chemicals migrate out of products and into the home environment, sticking to other surfaces. The products that are most concerning are the ones we touch every day: foam mattresses, pillows, and bedding (sheets and blankets). An excellent resource for organic bedding is the Clean Bedroom (www.thecleanbedroom.com).

Foam items manufactured in the United States and purchased after 2004 are unlikely to contain PBDEs because the chemical is now illegal to use. If you can't replace older items likely to contain PBDEs, you can still take these simple steps to reduce your exposure:

- **Inspect old foam:** Replace anything with a ripped cover or foam that is misshapen, visible, or breaking down.
- **Be careful when removing old carpet:** The padding may contain PBDEs. Isolate your work area from the rest of your home. Clean up with a HEPA-filter vacuum and mop to pick up as many of the small particles as possible. Remove all scrap foam from your home and yard immediately.
- **Avoid PBDEs in electronics:** One form of PBDE known as deca-BDE is still used in computer and television monitors and other electronic products, including mobile phones, fax machines, remote controls, video equipment, printers, photocopiers, toner cartridges,

and scanners. It can also be found in kitchen appliances, fans, heaters or hair dryers, water heaters, and lamp sockets. To reduce exposure, I suggest that you use these products in well-ventilated areas of your home, and if they are damaged or malfunctioning in any way, replace them with a new model.

Electrical Pollution

There is another form of pollution that you cannot see, taste, or smell and is neither chemical nor biological: electromagnetic pollution. "Dirty electricity," essentially poor power quality, refers to a combination of harmonics and transients generated primarily by electronic devices and especially by nonlinear loads like wireless devices. As we've become increasingly wired, it has become ever-present in homes.

Our reliance on electronic devices and wireless technology is contributing to an unprecedented increase in our exposure to a broad range of electromagnetic frequencies. This energy is generally categorized into two groups: low-frequency electric power (measured up to sixty hertz) and high-frequency wireless electronic devices (measured as megahertz and gigahertz). Electric pollution occurs from overexposure to a variety of electric sources, including power lines, computers, plasma TVs, dimmer switches, energy efficient lighting, cordless phones, personal electronic devices, wireless routers, or nearby cell phone and broadcast antennas.

Accumulated exposure to the electromagnetic field can affect health, causing electrical hypersensitivity. Symptoms can include fatigue, aches and pains, headaches, sleep disturbances, depression, anxiety, digestive problems, memory loss, difficulty concentrating, tremors, and tingling in the extremities. A 2008 study published in *Electromagnetic Biology and Medicine* suggested that electric pollution can even elevate blood sugar in sensitive diabetics.

Solutions: You can turn off your cell phone and MP3 player and unplug other electronic devices when not in use: not only will you reduce your exposure to dirty electricity; you'll save on your energy bill as well. Devices for determining if your home or workplace is exposed to dirty electricity can be found at Stetzer Electric (www.stetzerelectric.com).

Heavy Metal Exposure in the Home

We have already used the term "heavy metal" several times, particularly in connection with mercury and lead. Heavy metals are naturally occurring compounds, minerals, or elements that have always been here. They are liberated during mining and industrial processes, and the burning of fossil fuels also releases heavy metals, so they are spread even by the exhaust from our cars. Many of the particles are very small and can travel long distances. Heavy metals are now found in our soil, air, water, and food.

Many heavy metals are harmful to plants, animals, and humans because metals interfere with normal cellular functions. When even low levels of heavy metals accumulate in the body, they cause dysfunction. For example, the body holds on to mercury and lead because chemically they both look a great deal like the beneficial minerals zinc, selenium, and magnesium. These minerals are necessary to engage certain enzymes that are involved with every physiological process, including making sex hormones, balancing immune system function, and creating cellular energy. But the heavy metals block these good minerals from doing their jobs properly, thereby causing toxicity.

The most common heavy metals are arsenic, cadmium, lead, and mercury. My practice is located in New York City, and I've found that my patients with heavy metal sensitivities or allergies are typically affected by lead and mercury, which may be toxic even at trace levels.

Lead in Your Home Can Affect You

Any house built before 1978 may contain lead paint and lead plumbing. I've even treated patients with lead toxicity from eating off lead-glazed pottery (even retailers like Pottery Barn have been implicated because of imported pottery glazed outside the United States). Sixty percent of lead is used in the manufacturing of batteries (automobile batteries in particular), while the remainder is used in the production of pigments, glazes, solder, plastics, cable sheathing, ammunition, weights, gasoline additives, and a variety of other products. Lead crystal has lead in it and so does bronze. The industries that produce these products continue to pose a significant health risk to their workers and surrounding communities.

Lead is a neurological toxin that can affect your thinking and cognition. Symptoms of lead poisoning include learning disabilities, behavioral problems, reduced IQ, mental retardation, academic failure, and brain damage. When lead levels are very high, it can cause seizure, coma, and even death. Lead is also a tissue toxin that has been implicated as a cause of high blood pressure as well as kidney disease in older men and women.

Our bodies store lead in bone. As we get older, the bone starts breaking down and the lead is re-released into the body. Many postmenopausal women develop high blood pressure because once they stop producing hormones their bones start releasing lead into their blood.

If you live in an older home, simply painting over old lead paint is not enough to prevent exposure. Eventually, latex paints will peel off older lead surfaces. Old lead paint has a unique look: tiny cracks run through it in parallel lines and then little connectors divide it, almost like a honeycomb. You can buy test strips at your local hardware store to confirm the lead content of your home. If the levels are high, a professional can remove the paint without exposing the rest of your home.

Mercury Is Pervasive

Elemental mercury, the kind found in thermometers, blood pressure cuffs, lamps, and dental amalgams (silver fillings), is responsible for the least common form of acute poisoning because it is poorly absorbed into the body. However, small amounts of elemental mercury can vaporize at room temperature or with friction, including the act of chewing in someone with many mercury dental amalgams, and then it can be swallowed and converted to the very toxic methylmercury (organic mercury) by intestinal bacteria. Over time, this low-level exposure may accumulate in your body causing neurologic and immune system dysfunction. When methylmercury is absorbed into the bloodstream, it can be toxic to the organs and the central nervous system.

Inorganic mercury, found in lamps, wood preservatives, disinfectants, explosives, inks, cosmetics, and various chemical products, is absorbed both orally and through the skin, and is usually responsible for acute mercury poisoning with central nervous system symptoms.

Ethyl mercury is found as thimerosal, a common medical preservative.

Mercury is found in the following household items:

- coal-burning stoves (elemental mercury)
- fluorescent lightbulbs (elemental mercury)
- hair dyes (ethyl mercury)

Products containing mercury, like thermometers and fluorescent lightbulbs, must be disposed of properly. They cannot be thrown into the home garbage because if they are broken the mercury vapors will spread into the environment. Instead, these items need to be brought to a recycling or disposal center. You can contact your local municipal waste agency directly or go to the EPA Web site (www.epa.gov/bulbrecycling) or Earth911.com (www.earth911.com) to identify local recycling options.

Mercury Can Be an Allergen *and* a Toxin

There are two main health issues surrounding mercury: toxicity and allergy. It is well established in the scientific and medical literature that mercury has a significant impact on proper cellular function. It is considered toxic because it interferes with the ability of minerals found within the body to activate receptors on the enzymes within our cells that are necessary for body functions like creating energy, creating brain chemicals, and even creating proper immune system responses.

Imagine sticking the wrong key into a lock. Even though the key fits, it can't open the door and, worse, if it breaks off inside the lock, no matter how much you want to open the door with the correct key, the lock is jammed, making the room inaccessible. This is exactly how mercury causes cellular toxicity: it prevents our cells from activating or deactivating primary processes. For example, mercury can block the ability of the mineral selenium to activate immune and antioxidant enzymes, thereby making us more susceptible to infections and allergies.

Additionally, mercury can cause an allergic reaction, a type of autoimmune disease. It is known to cause people to have rashes, hives, and even a lupus-like autoimmune reaction. Other heavy metals are known to cause rashes. For example, when some people wear nickel, which is commonly used in jewelry, belt buckles, and buttons, they can get rashes. These people are having an allergic reaction to nickel. The same thing can happen when a person has mercury fillings in their teeth: they can have an immune system reaction to the fillings in their mouth. The American Dental Association suspects that as much as 5 percent of the population may have a mercury allergy.

If mercury fillings are removed, many times this will eliminate the allergy symptoms. However, if mercury has accumulated in the body tissue, that mercury must be gotten rid of as well. The main way the body is able to dispose of heavy metals in the tissue is through its own detoxification system, which relies on metallothionein, a chelating or binding protein produced in the body, along with the cellular antioxidant glutathione and the minerals zinc, selenium, and magnesium. These compounds and minerals work together to absorb the mercury and other heavy metals, and then inactivate them and transport them out of the body. However, when the body's detoxification system gets overloaded, heavy metals, like any other toxin, can't leave the body easily, which is why we have to augment the detoxification process with supplements, saunas, or prescription binding agents like dimercapto-succinic acid (DMSA).

CADMIUM IS FOUND IN COSTUME JEWELRY

Miley Cyrus brand bracelets, charms, and necklaces sold exclusively at Walmart stores were pulled off the shelves in 2010 because they contained high levels of the toxic heavy metal cadmium. The items are not known to be dangerous if they are simply worn, but concerns arose because the young girls who bought the items might suck on, bite, or inadvertently swallow them. Long-term exposure to cadmium can lead to bone softening and kidney failure as well as cancer.

Katherine Was Allergic to Mercury

I first met Katherine when she was twenty-nine years old. She came to my office because she was experiencing a significant decrease in appetite along with weight loss, fatigue, and itchy rashes all over her body. She had been seen by a local dermatologist who, after performing a blood mercury test and a DMSA chelation challenge, recognized that she had elevated mercury levels in her tissue. Yet after three months of treatment with a prescription binding agent, DMSA, plus instructions to avoid eating fish thought to be high in mercury, there was no noticeable improvement in her symptoms.

When I saw her in my office, I tried to look for another source of mercury in her life. After a thorough medical evaluation, I told Katherine that she might be allergic to her mercury fillings, which could cause her to have skin reactions and contribute to her chronic fatigue. After a great deal of conversation and weighing of the risks, benefits, and alternatives to treatment, we concluded that she should have her fillings evaluated and replaced with nonmetal composite fillings. Since she only had a few, this was not a difficult task. Sure enough, after she had all her mercury fillings removed her rash disappeared and her energy, memory, and itchiness all improved significantly.

Two years later Katherine came back to see me. She was concerned that she was not able to become pregnant after a full year of unsuccessful attempts. Within three months of working together to improve her body's detoxification process, she came back into the office. This time she was elated to report that she was pregnant.

Katherine is a great example of how mercury can disrupt the immune system and, in this case, cause an allergic reaction. It also shows that when you are able to improve your innate detoxification process, the rest of your body responds positively as well. In Katherine's case, her body naturally became a hospitable place for childbearing.

Choosing the Right Plastics

Recyclable plastics are marked with numbers 1–7. Look for these numbers on the bottom of plastic bottles and plastic containers. Based on current research, only numbers 1, 2, 4, and 5 are considered acceptable. These plastics have the lowest risk of leaching into food and water.

Items marked with the number 7 should be avoided. Number 7 is a catchall category that includes the new safer bioplastics made from sugarcane and corn but also unsafe BPA plastic. Plastics marked 3 are polyvinyl chloride (PVC) plastics used to make food wrap, bottles for cooking oil, and plumbing pipes. They contain phthalates, which can be released into food when the plastic is heated. Polystyrene (Styrofoam) plastics are numbered 6 and used to make disposable containers, plates, and cups. Evidence suggests that toxic chemicals leach into food when it is heated, so it is best to avoid this plastic as much as possible and to only drink cold liquids from them.

The following plastics are considered safest:

- Number 1 (polyethylene terephthalate/ethylene, or PET/PETE) plastics are used for plastic water bottles and are probably acceptable for one-time use. Do not let them overheat and do not reuse them, because they have a porous surface that allows bacteria to accumulate over time.

- Number 2 (high-density polyethylene, or HDPE) plastics are usually opaque and are used for milk jugs, detergent bottles, and juice bottles.
- Number 4 (low-density polyethylene, or LDPE) plastics are used for plastic bags, food storage, some food wraps, and squeezable bottles.
- Number 5 (polypropylene, or PP) plastics are used for yogurt cups, ketchup and syrup bottles, and straws.

Additionally, even plastics that are considered microwave safe are not my first choice for heating foods. They are considered microwave safe because they don't melt in the microwave, not because they are safe for our food or for us. Instead use glass or ceramic containers that are free of metallic paint. Avoid using plastics for storing fatty foods, as there is greater leaching of chemicals into fatty foods. Also beware of cling wraps, especially for microwave use. Instead use waxed paper or paper towels for covering foods.

If you must use plastic in the microwave or to wrap foods, don't let the plastic touch the food. Either wrap the food in a paper towel first, and then wrap with plastic, or slice off a thin layer where the food came in contact with the plastic and rewrap it in non-PVC plastic wrap or place it in a container.

I do not recommend the use of plastic water bottles. If you must, choose polycarbonate bottles, to reduce leaching of BPA, and do not use them for warm or hot liquids. Discard old or scratched bottles. Water bottles made from number 1 or 2 plastics should only be used once and not be refilled.

You can reduce bacterial contamination of all types of plastic by thoroughly washing them daily. However, avoid using harsh detergents that can break down the plastic and increase chemical leaching.

PLANTS HELP REDUCE POLLUTION, INDOORS AND OUT

One natural way to help lower volatile organic chemicals in your home environment is as easy as bringing in houseplants. Spider plants or broad leaf plants like snake plants are known for having great air-cleansing ability. Also consider ficus, peace lily, Chinese evergreen, and heart-leaf philodendron.

Instead of turning to harsh chemicals, you can plant flowers and herbs in your garden to keep bugs away. These plants can also help to enrich your soil. For example, planting garlic alongside roses or lettuce will keep aphids, Japanese beetles, and spider mites at bay. Planting mint near tomatoes deters all kinds of pests, including ants, fleas, and even rodents. And pretty nasturtium flowers growing under fruit trees will keep aphids from nibbling.

Mold Is a Toxic Health Concern

Molds are fungi that reproduce by releasing tiny spores into the air. The spores that land on moist objects begin to grow and develop. There are thousands of different types of mold, which can be found both outside and inside your home and on any potentially damp surface, including the human body. Molds can look like a brown stain or black spots, like what you typically find in a shower stall. Other times they can appear in different colors, including green, yellow, or red, and each color signals a different type of mold organism.

If there is water damage or standing water in your home—in a shower or bathtub, for example—mold has the potential to grow. It will attach itself to water-damaged wood or grow underneath flooring tile or carpeting and even on furniture. When it grows to a certain level, it can produce enough spores and potentially toxic products to eventually make you sick.

The most common molds found in the home are penicillium, aspergillus, and cladosporium. Floating particles of mold are invisible to the naked eye, so it's impossible to see where they will land until they begin to grow. Loose mold particles are easily inhaled and can be a constant irritation. When mold is growing excessively in your home, you can experience symptoms like itchy eyes, chronic stuffy nose, itchy ears, and skin rashes: these are generally considered to be allergic reactions to mold or mold spores.

However, if you start having more severe symptoms of mold exposure, such as difficulty concentrating, irritability, brain fog, or memory changes, these could be related to the toxic mold stachybotrys, which not only produces spores but also mold toxins that affect the nervous system. Toxic mold is a type of mold that produces hazardous neurotoxin by-products called mycotoxins. These mycotoxins are more likely to trigger health problems in otherwise healthy individuals. Stachybotrys is a slimy, greenish black mold that grows on moisture-laden materials that contain cellulose, such as wood, paper, or drywall. It does not grow on tile or cement.

Evaluating Your Home for Mold

There are two phases to test for mold toxins or allergens: you need to test yourself as well as your home. Simple blood and allergy tests at the doctor's office will confirm if you have a true mold allergy. There are also test kits that can evaluate the condition of the mold in your home. The tests involve a culture medium that is placed where mold growth is high or likely to be high. You can also hire an environmental remediation company to come into your home and take spot cultures or ventilation tests. Even if the mold in your home is not toxic, it can still affect your health and degrade your indoor air quality.

Once you determine that you have mold growing in your home, and your skin or blood testing confirms that you are allergic or sensitive to the mold, the next step is to remove it and eliminate the sources of exposure. While mold is a problem, in most instances its growth can be prevented or stopped before it causes excessive damage. First, you have to make sure that the water damage has been corrected. This might mean that plumbing or other leakages into the home have to be addressed as well as the surfaces that contain the mold.

The next step is removing the mold, which might require replacing drywall, floorboards and other flooring materials (carpeting, tile), re-caulking along shower and bath areas, or re-grouting brick. It is possible to clean away mold without adding to your body burden by using harsh chemicals. Make sure the room is well ventilated before you begin. Allow the space or surface to dry completely, and then apply a solution of one-half cup bleach per gallon of water to help kill the remaining mold and spores.

MOLD GROWS INSIDE US

Mold symptoms can occur when there is mold literally growing in a body that is out of balance. Toenail fungus, athlete's foot, and ringworm are all different types of mold that grow on our skin when our body isn't healthy. It's also possible to have mold growing in your sinuses, ears, and even in the digestive tract. If mold is growing in or on you, it is a sign that there is some other imbalance in the body that needs to be corrected.

Mold thrives in damp conditions:

- Bathrooms with poor ventilation
- Clothes dryers and exhaust fans that vent under the house or back into the room
- Leaks from the outdoors into the home
- Water pipes

Stop mold growth by:

- Covering crawlspace dirt with plastic and ensuring that the area is well ventilated

- Adding storm windows to eliminate condensation on glass
- Installing dehumidifiers in chronically moist rooms
- Insulating pipes and other cold surfaces to discourage condensation
- Removing carpets from rooms that stay damp

Will Was Sensitive to Mold

Mold symptoms are very similar to other medical problems. For example, I once had a patient, Will, who came to see me with achy muscles, achy joints, fatigue, and difficulty concentrating. Will believed that he had Lyme disease because he frequently vacationed in upstate New York and the Hamptons, where Lyme disease is endemic. What's more, many of his friends have had similar symptoms relating to Lyme disease. However, one particular aspect of his symptoms made me think twice about his self-diagnosis. He told me that his symptoms would always get worse when he was at work and seemed to disappear when he went on vacation out of the country.

After Will filled out the detox questionnaire and completed a thorough physical exam, I ordered the appropriate blood work for Lyme disease as well as immunologic testing for standard allergies, including mold. The results showed that Will did not have Lyme, but his allergy levels for molds were significantly elevated.

I then sent Will to do a thorough evaluation of his home and work environment. In a few days, he was able to trace his symptoms to a ventilation duct that was contaminated with mold. The duct emptied contaminated air over his work desk every single day. This was the reason why Will felt better when he was away from the office for long periods of time.

Once we found the source of the mold, resolving his symptoms was relatively easy. Will followed the detox diet for thirty days. He avoided sugar, bread, beer, and wine, which are all foods that can aggravate internal yeast symptoms. At the same time, his office cleaned the ventilation duct that emptied over his desk. He also began using a HEPA filter at home and in the office, switched from antibacterial soap to glycerin soap, and stopped using plastic to store or microwave food. After his thorough detox, and instructions on keeping his home and office free of mold, Will felt great, and continues to do so.

This chapter covered many different ways for you to detox your home. By following these suggestions, you'll lower your sources of exposure and your body burden, which may automatically alleviate some of your symptoms even before you start the diet modifications.

Here are some simple solutions that you can follow. The more you employ, the healthier you and your environment will become:

- Use a HEPA filter at home or work. A good resource is the E. L. Foust Company (www.foustco.com).
- Use natural home-cleaning products.
- Cook with Pyrex, cooking-grade stainless steel, or old-fashioned cast-iron cookware.
- Select 100 percent natural skin care products and check for unsafe ingredients on EWG's online database (www.cosmeticsdatabase .com).
- Avoid PBDE fire retardants.
- Turn off power switches and unplug infrequently used equipment and home appliances.
- Be aware of and limit sources of lead and mercury in your home and environment.
- Only use the safest plastics: numbers 1, 2, 4, and 5.
- Never eat food from heated plastic, regardless of whether it is considered microwave safe.
- Keep plants in your home; they are natural air filters.
- Maintain dry home conditions to prevent mold growth.

Chapter 5

Is Your Diet Making You Sick?

Whether you eat fresh, preserved, or processed foods that are coated with pesticide residue, or enjoy a highly refined diet that is loaded with sugar, or fill up with lots of bread and pasta, which typically don't have tons of vitamins and minerals, you are exposing your body to potentially toxic chemicals. An unhealthy or nutritiously incomplete diet can literally make you sick.

Even though youth has its advantages, it also has a large disadvantage when it comes to toxic exposure. Younger people have been growing up with food that is generally considered to be less nutritious. And, the foods we eat now are potentially more toxic because of exposures to pesticides, insecticides, preservatives, and hormones. The younger you are, the more likely it is that your entire diet has been compromised, giving you a greater uninterrupted exposure to these chemicals.

For years food manufacturers and marketers have put their emphasis on products with long shelf lives rather than on nutritional value, so they sell food products that are loaded with chemical preservatives, guaranteeing consistency of taste and an unimaginably long time before they go bad. The preservatives used are meant to limit the growth of bacteria and mold on refined foods. Yet as a result, you may be eating foods that even bacteria and mold do not want to eat.

Worse, while you are enjoying these low-nutrient and potentially hazardous foods, you aren't getting the nutrition your body requires, making it more difficult to maintain an optimal level of health. Your body will have to struggle to sustain its most important organ systems—like the heart and the brain—in order to keep them working properly. Sometimes this occurs at the expense of other body functions, including your body's innate detoxification system: the liver, kidneys, and immune system.

The signs that your body is not getting enough nutrient-rich foods or is being exposed to too many unhealthy chemicals in the form of pesticides, preservatives, or additives include fatigue, difficulty concentrating, achiness, muscle twitches, rashes, inflammation, chronic colds, and skin infections. As you can see, many of these are the same signs and symptoms linked to toxic exposures. That's one of the reasons why I believe that the high-sugar foods, processed dairy products, and white grains in the standard American diet are just as toxic to the body as environmental pollutants.

How Your Body Suffers

After prolonged exposure to a toxic diet, the digestive tract eventually loses the good bacteria necessary to digest and help absorb nutrients properly. Bad bacteria or yeast begin to colonize the colon. This change causes food to ferment in the intestines, creating gas and bloating. Worse, the new bacteria and yeast aren't recognized by the immune system, 70 percent of which is located in the digestive tract. Instead, the bacteria and yeast are considered foreign, stimulating an immune system response and causing inflammation in the digestive tract, which leads to a breakdown in the normal structure of the intestines.

The inflammation widens the junctions between the cells of the intestinal lining, allowing incompletely digested particles of food to be partially absorbed. This is called leaky gut syndrome. These particles are then targeted by antibodies, forming immune complexes, which cause a chronic, semi-infectious state and can be spread by the bloodstream to the rest of the body. Low-grade fever and inconsistent gut pain are common complaints of patients with leaky gut syndrome.

The body tries to adapt to regular exposure to improperly digested foods by regulating its immune response. I like to compare this response to the way firefighters react to a forest fire that starts to burn out of control. Firefighters are taught to respond severely, swiftly, and without hesitation to even the slightest threat. Unfortunately, their actions cause a great deal of collateral damage. In the case of your immune system, it becomes hyperstimulated by the exposure to improperly digested foods, and you may find that your immune response is suddenly aroused and that you are more susceptible to seasonal allergies, rashes, or even auto-immune diseases like rheumatoid arthritis, systemic lupus, or Hashimoto's thyroiditis.

If the immune system continues to be overstimulated for a long period, a different, unregulated immune response can occur. This time the immune system loses its normal control mechanisms. Imagine that the firefighters, acting without the oversight of a chief, start searching every home in the city for fires. Obviously, this is a very poor use of resources because when a real fire springs up all the firemen will be already occupied with this futile search. When the immune system is unregulated, it reacts to every exposure, whether threatening or not. Eventually, this can cause chemical sensitivities and make a person sensitive to all environmental exposures. Worse, it may lead to cancer because the immune system is just too overwhelmed and burned out to react appropriately to abnormally developing cells.

Food Allergies Are Toxins

Often the foods you most frequently eat will become the most toxic to your system. You might find that you experience these symptoms whenever you are exposed to even the tiniest amount of particular foods. In short, these foods have become toxic to your body. Your immune system identifies those foods as being foreign and creates an immune response in the form of an allergic reaction, which can include a rash, hives, stuffy nose, watery eyes, vomiting, choking, coughing, asthma, or external inflammation (e.g., swollen hands or face). In severe situations, you can develop internal swelling that can lead to anaphylaxis: a deadly condition where the throat closes so that air cannot pass through to the lungs.

A food allergy is generally defined as an immediate immune system response to eating that food. Also called an IgE-related allergy, this immune response can generally be confirmed with a blood test. The number of people with true IgE-related food allergies is small. The most likely culprits for IgE-related food allergies include wheat, dairy products, soy, eggs, oranges, strawberries, and peanuts. My suspicion is that people have difficulties with these particular foods because they tend to be highly refined, genetically modified, or heavily treated with pesticides.

The only way to avoid having an IgE-related allergic reaction is to identify which foods you are allergic to, and then completely avoid eating or touching them. Some allergists and environmental medicine doctors, like me, may treat individuals with IgE-related food allergies with a desensitization program, which involves a series of injections that expose the individual to microscopic amounts of the food they are allergic to so that the immune system will retrain itself to accept these foods as friendly instead of foreign. However, I always prefer patients to do the best they can to simply avoid the foods.

Food Sensitivities Are Different from Allergies

Your body can also have another exaggerated immune response to foods, causing a second type of problem known as "food sensitivity." This is classified as an IgG4-mediated or delayed type of food response. When this occurs, you will notice that you are more susceptible to chronic recurring colds and infections, and you may have difficulties recovering from viruses like mononucleosis. You may also find that you develop sensitivities to other environmental exposures, like the smell of fragrances, gasoline, new furniture, or even new carpeting. These symptoms can be a sign that you are beginning to develop environmental sensitivity, a situation in which your immune system is burned out.

Food sensitivities look completely different from food allergies, yet they are just as difficult to deal with. First, food sensitivity is usually a delayed reaction: the body may not respond to the problematic food for up to seventy-two hours after it is consumed. This means that you may have a reaction to a food you eat today as many as three days later. Unfortunately, this makes it difficult to relate a particular food to a reaction in the body. Consequently, not all doctors believe that food sensitivities exist. However, in my practice I have seen the profound changes that can take place in a patient's health after they avoid and eliminate the offending foods from their diet.

The symptoms of an IgG4 food sensitivity reaction are typically not the same as those of an allergic reaction. Instead of an inflammatory response, you may experience more subtle changes to your health, including low energy, cold symptoms, difficulty concentrating, digestive gas, bloating, fluid retention, or weight gain. Yet food sensitivities are still considered to be an immune response. If food sensitivity is not identified early, the body can develop a response that becomes more severe each time the culprit-food is consumed.

This constant exposure can eventually develop into an autoimmune response. For example, people with sensitivity to the wheat protein gluten are more likely to have other autoimmune diseases like rheumatoid arthritis or Hashimoto's thyroiditis. The longer the person goes without recognizing the food sensitivity, the more likely it is that the person will develop a more severe autoimmune disease or some other health problem. However, if the foods causing the problems can be identified and eliminated early enough, then the immune system can heal itself. The good news is that generally food sensitivities do not turn into food allergies.

Children and adults with food sensitivities may be susceptible to chronic throat or nasal infections. Many times the symptoms are treated as infections without determining the underlying cause. Long courses of antibiotics may be inappropriately prescribed, with only temporary improvement in symptoms. If you are being treated repeatedly with antibiotics without resolution of your symptoms, you may have an underlying food sensitivity. If the culprit-food is removed, your recurring infections should disappear.

People commonly develop sensitivities to the same foods that cause allergic reactions. In addition, wheat, dairy products, and sugar are particularly detrimental. These are generally the most processed and refined foods in a typical diet. In addition, dairy product consumption can increase mucus production, which can worsen seasonal allergies and colds. Wheat and sugar are both highly processed and can actually cause fermentation of yeast in the digestive tract, causing symptoms of abdominal gas and bloating, and even a hangover effect, after eating too much sugar or wheat. You'll learn more about these three food groups later in this chapter and why you'll need to eliminate all of them during your detox.

For Some, Gluten Is Toxic

Gluten is a natural protein found in grains such as wheat, oats, barley, rye, and spelt. It also happens to be the protein that makes breads fluffy and chewy, and it's excellent for thickening sauces, making dough sticky, and enhancing the shelf life of breads, cookies, and cakes, all of which are advantages in the consumer marketplace. During the process of "improving" the commercial applications of wheat grain, the U.S. agricultural industry increased its gluten content through hybridization and genetic selection. With each year of crop growth, they identified the seeds of grains that had the highest gluten content and used only those seeds in the following planting seasons.

The wheat industry was widely successful in its quest to enhance gluten content. However, gluten turns out to be highly irritating to the immune system and an allergenic substance for many people. When the gluten content of grains was low, people susceptible to gluten sensitivity would rarely experience an immune system reaction because the amount they were exposed to was below the threshold their immune system had for being irritated. Yet in the past twenty to twenty-five years, since the hybridization occurred, the gluten content of wheat in the United States has increased between 30 and 50 percent, and thus people who were on the cusp of having a gluten sensitivity started having immune reactions.

What's more, the immune reaction associated with gluten is not limited to digestive symptoms: gluten sensitivity can affect any part of the body. In his pivotal book *Dangerous Grains*, Dr. James Braly alerted the medical community to the fact that the immune response to gluten affects more than just the digestive tract, as it does with celiac disease. It is also linked to chronic sinus infections, ear infections, joint problems, skin rashes, and memory changes. One of the reasons why some children who are sensitive to gluten develop severe behavioral disturbances is that they cannot completely digest the gluten protein, and the excess amount becomes absorbed in the body as a morphine-like compound called gluteomorphin, which can be irritating to the nervous system.

Interestingly, many of my patients with gluten sensitivity do not have difficulties with glutenous foods when they travel outside the country, particularly to Europe. There they can eat bread, pasta, cookies, and cakes, generally without any type of reaction. This is because those grains have not been hybridized and have much less gluten. Meanwhile, the U.S. government is working with the World Health Organization to introduce the hybridized grain as the standard throughout the world.

You can test to see if you have gluten sensitivity by following the elimination diet described below. You will eliminate glutenous foods from your diet for a period of time—ranging from one week to four weeks—then reintroduce them into your diet and see if you have a reaction. Additionally, a medical doctor can perform a variety of diagnostic blood tests, including antigliadin antibody, anti-endomysial antibody, and transglutaminase antibody tests. However, to correctly diagnose celiac disease a colonoscopy must be ordered to take a sample of tissue from the intestinal mucosa.

Where Gluten Is Found

To avoid gluten, avoid food and drinks containing the following:

- barley
- bulgur
- durum
- farina
- graham flour
- Kamut (Khorasan wheat)
- malt
- matzo meal
- rye
- semolina
- spelt
- triticale
- wheat

Avoid these foods entirely unless labeled "gluten free":

- beer
- bread
- cake
- candy
- cereal
- cookies
- couscous
- crackers
- croutons
- gravy

- imitation meats or seafood
- oats
- pasta
- pie
- processed luncheon meats
- soy sauce
- salad dressing
- self-basting poultry

Other products that may contain gluten include:

- food additives, such as malt flavoring
- lipsticks and lip balms
- medications and vitamins that use gluten as a binding agent
- toothpaste

Foods allowed in a gluten-free diet include the following:

- amaranth
- arrowroot
- buckwheat
- corn and cornmeal
- gluten-free flours (rice, potato, bean)
- hominy grits
- millet
- polenta
- quinoa
- rice
- sweet potatoes
- tapioca
- vegetables
- wine and distilled nongluten grain liquors (e.g., single-ingredient potato vodkas like Chopin vodka or Luksusowa vodka) or tequila

Thomas Was Incorrectly Diagnosed with Schizophrenia

One of my most eye-opening experiences in using the detox diet was with my patient Thomas. Tom was barely making ends meet because he'd been placed on work disability after being diagnosed with schizophrenia. This psychological condition impairs a person's ability to perceive the difference between what is real and what is not real. Tom came to see me for nutritional counseling and suggestions on what nutritional modifications he might follow to improve his symptoms.

As part of his workup, Thomas filled out the detox questionnaire, and I was shocked to see that his total score was 140 (remember, the goal is 14 or below). I recommended that we immediately check his blood levels for food allergies, nutritional deficiencies, and a variety of toxins, and while he was waiting for the results, I suggested that he start the detox diet.

After just four weeks on the diet, he returned to my office and told me that he felt so good that he would be able to return to work within the coming month. He completed a new detox questionnaire, and we were both pleased to see that his total score had dropped to 28. What's more, I told Tom that his blood work showed that he had severe gluten intolerance. I explained that because he was on the detox diet he was already avoiding gluten, but that he should continue to avoid it for the rest of his life. He was very happy to do so, seeing how much better he felt physically and mentally. Now he understood the underlying cause of his symptoms.

The Detox Diet: Identifying Your Food Issues

Like Thomas, you can experience a complete reversal of many of your symptoms just by eliminating foods that are toxic to your system. When you stop eating the most likely culprits all at once, your digestive and immune systems have a chance to rest, heal, and reset. Then, once the elimination diet is completed and those foods are reintroduced one by one, you'll be able to determine which ones are causing your health issues.

An elimination diet is considered the "gold standard," the best way of determining what foods are causing sensitivities or allergies. No blood test or skin test works as well. The only drawback to the diet is that it is time-consuming. Each food group that you eliminate needs to be introduced back into the diet one at a time. If you resume eating a type of food and feel fine—do not experience any symptoms—then you are not sensitive to that food and can probably continue eating it without any problems. However, if you add a type of food and begin to notice symptoms, such as fatigue or fluid retention or whatever symptom you had before, then that food will have to be eliminated for at least three months, if not longer, in an attempt to fully reset your immune system to accommodate that particular type of food.

Another benefit to doing the detox diet is that you will not only feel better, but you will also find that you are able to lose a significant amount of weight. By avoiding the foods you are sensitive to, you are producing less internal inflammation, which means you will be able to get rid of the fluid and fat you have unwittingly been holding on to. My patients also are thrilled to report that their skin begins to look better, they have fewer seasonal allergies, and they feel calm and clearheaded. As you cleanse your body, you'll clear your mind.

Foods You Will Eliminate

The goal of any elimination diet is to identify and avoid sources of toxic exposure.

Some food groups are eliminated specifically for health reasons that are not environmentally related. Others are environmentally related. The foods you'll be avoiding may be slowing down the detoxification process. For example, dairy products create mucus in some people, which slows down detoxification and is why you'll be eliminating it for the next few weeks.

You'll also avoid processed foods such as refined sugar, bread, pasta, cookies, candies, and cakes. Processed foods are loaded with chemicals and preservatives. Even organic versions of these products that do not contain chemicals need to be eliminated. That's because the dietary culprit that contributes most frequently to various diseases and inflammation is refined sugar, which is found in most processed foods.

Processed foods can also directly affect your health by causing insulin resistance. Processed carbohydrates break down and are absorbed into the blood too quickly, causing a spike in blood sugar. The body responds by spiking its own insulin levels, and, over time, every cell in our body develops a resistance. This is just like a manual laborer who, over time, develops calluses on their hands from many days of hard work. The calluses provide protection from the repetitive stress of labor, at the cost of having less sensitivity in the hands. When that happens on a cellular level, we lose our sensitivity to insulin, which is the first step to metabolic dysfunction and diabetes. By following the elimination detox diet, you'll begin the process of resting your cells and allowing them to heal and become sensitive, which for some people can actually reverse the course toward diabetes.

Avoid Sugar

Sugar is loaded into desserts and treats and has also found its way into main courses. Manufacturers add sugar to everything: it is one of the two primary food additives—the other is salt—used to enhance the taste of processed foods, from breakfast cereals to pasta sauce to soups. Sugar has such an intense flavor that it literally stuns our ability to taste other things.

Sugar is made by a variety of plants as a way to store energy they don't need; just like we store energy or extra calories as body fat. Each year 120 million tons of refined sugar is produced, 70 percent from sugarcane and 30 percent from beets. Processed sugar really has no health benefits and no nutritional content, especially after it's been refined. When it starts out as sugarcane, it actually has some nutritional value, but when processed, it, just like any refined food, loses its nutritional value and becomes highly potent. The sugarcane or beets go through a multistage refining process to remove impurities, nutrients, and color, leaving a very clean, white product. Brown sugar and "sugar in the raw" are nothing more than refined sugar with caramel-colored syrup added.

The end product is sweet and extremely addictive. If you are a "sugar junkie," you'll recognize the sign of addiction: every time you have sugar you may need a little more to get the feeling of satisfaction you crave. The reason sugar is so much more addictive than sweet fruit is because it's highly purified and concentrated, just like the illegal drug crack is much more addictive than the cocaine it comes from. And like any other addiction, weaning yourself off sugar can be difficult. Many of my patients have told me that they experienced withdrawal symptoms during the first week of the elimination diet. Don't worry: the symptoms disappear quickly. And best of all, the cravings for sugar don't return.

While sugar doesn't affect the way your body processes toxins, over-exposure to it increases your likelihood of developing diabetes. It also stuns your immune system, making it less active against infections. Sugar will stun white blood cells for about ten minutes after it's consumed. It also causes the hormones in the body to become out of balance, as is the case with spiking insulin levels. Insulin is a growth hormone as well as a shepherd for herding sugar into cells. If your body is constantly getting sugar and insulin spikes, then it is constantly getting the signal to grow. But instead of getting taller, the growth is in fat cells.

The body tries to maintain balance, or homeostasis, of blood sugar, but with constant spiking, we begin to feel it when our blood sugar drops, which is called hypoglycemia. This puts the body into a stress response where it is forced to create sugar on its own by producing the hormones glucagon and adrenaline. That's why when you eat a high-sugar meal you initially feel a burst of energy but then feel tired afterward when the blood sugar tries to stabilize. You may also feel irritable or unfocused. This happens when the body is producing adrenaline, the fight-or-flight hormone, which triggers the body to seek out more food to get into balance again, at almost any cost. You many find that many of your emotional problems, including anxiousness, depression, and irritability will dissipate during the elimination diet because you won't be riding the sugar roller coaster all day long.

Sodas are loaded with sugars, so they will be avoided during the detox. Diet sodas are no better because of the artificial sweeteners. Despite the fact that artificial sweeteners have no calories, researchers have shown that they still stimulate insulin production. You'll also be limiting your alcohol, especially beer and wine because they are high in sugar. I recommend that you stay off the hard stuff for the duration of the elimination diet, but if you really must imbibe, limit yourself to no more than two vodka drinks a week.

Avoid Grains and Bread

Just like sugar, grains are commonly put through a multistage refining process during which the fiber, vitamins, minerals, and nutrients are removed until the final product is a white powder. Enriched flour is basically this powder with fiber, color, and vitamins and minerals added back into it.

Once you complete the elimination diet and determine that you can tolerate grains, you can make an informed decision about grains. If you really want to eat them, choose whole unrefined grains like quinoa, buckwheat, or Irish oats rather than pasta, rice, or couscous (which sounds exotic but is really just tiny balls of pasta). If you decide to eat bread, choose whole-grain bread instead of whole wheat. Whole wheat bread is generally white bread with caramel color. Whole-grain breads are definitely a better choice, and sprouted-grain breads are even better. Ezekiel 4:9, a brand of sprouted-grain bread often found in supermarkets' frozen section, is what I recommend to my patients. Sprouted grains actually have a higher nutritional content that the original grain and can be easier to digest.

An interesting article published in the *European Journal of Clinical Nutrition* in 1997 showed that our primitive ancestors got only 1 percent of their calories from grains and that 99 percent of their calories were from fruits, vegetables, roots, beans, nuts, and animal protein. Today typically 59 percent of our calories come from refined grains, 18 percent from refined and artificial sugars or sweeteners, and only 23 percent from fruits, vegetables, beans, nuts, and animal protein. We've come a long way from the diets our ancestors ate, and while our modern eating habits may be convenient, they might not be representative of what we were designed to eat.

Avoid Dairy Products

Dairy products are problematic because science has turned otherwise healthy whole milk into another processed food. The net result is that milk has become an enriched beverage that happens to cause allergies and sensitivities for many people.

Milk is highly refined and what we buy at the grocery store is anything but "natural." To enhance or prolong the shelf life of milk products, they are put through two processes: pasteurization and homogenization. Pasteurization involves heating the milk to very high temperatures to kill off bacteria, thereby increasing shelf life. But during this process milk enzymes and vitamins are destroyed and milk proteins become denatured. Without the naturally occurring enzymes, milk can be more difficult to digest, especially for someone who has lactose intolerance, which is simply another way of describing the inability to digest milk sugars. Synthetic versions of the vitamins destroyed in the pasteurization process, including vitamins A and D, must be added back in. Because the shape and structure of the milk proteins change when they are denatured, many people have an adverse immune system response to them: the proteins are recognized as unwelcome foreign material and instigate an immune response that can develop into a milk allergy.

In the homogenization process, milk is driven through a series of filters that reduces the size of its fat globules and allows the milk fat to stay suspended rather that rising to the top and separating. The small fat globules make a more attractive product, but the downside is that homogenized milk is more likely to become rancid and create inflammation in the body.

Large-scale dairy farms have injected milking cows with hormones, including genetically engineered rBGH (recombinant bovine growth hormone), which is used to enhance milk production by increasing levels of IGF-1 (insulin-like growth factor 1). In Europe and Canada, rBGH is banned due to concerns that the IGF-1 found in cows and cow's milk can increase the risk of estrogen-related cancers, like breast cancer, in humans. If you can safely reintroduce dairy products into your diet after the elimination diet, choose products that are clearly labeled "organic" with "no rBGH" or other hormones.

Avoid Nightshade Vegetables

During the detox, I also recommend avoiding nightshade vegetables. These include tomatoes, white potatoes, eggplant, peppers, and tobacco. All of these contain chemicals called saponins that can increase digestive trackt permeability and leaky gut syndrome. Among the typical symptoms of nightshade sensitivity are joint pain and inflammation. It has been my experience that, while people do not always develop arthritis from the nightshade vegetables, they can gain weight because of the inflammation those vegetables can cause.

If you already know that you are allergic to certain fruits or vegetables, you should continue to avoid them. However, you should be aware that certain fruits are related to other environmental allergies. For example, if you have weed allergies avoid peaches and mangos. Bananas, grapes, and oranges are common allergenic fruits, and they also have high sugar contents, so they should not be eaten during the elimination diet.

More of the "No" List

Some additional foods you'll avoid on the detox diet include the following:

- **Coffee:** Not because of the caffeine but because of the acidity. The body's detoxification pathways work best in an alkaline environment.
- **Seeds:** Avoid for weight loss because of their fat content (30–50 percent of the calories from seeds comes from fat).
- **Nuts:** Avoid for weight loss because of the fat content (60–70 percent of the calories from nuts comes from fat) and also because they can be allergenic.
- **Soy:** Frequently genetically modified and can cause allergies in many people. This includes foods like tofu, tempeh, textured soy protein, soy sauce, soy milk, and, of course, whole soybeans (edamame). Soy is also used to make cereal, salad dressings, meat alternatives, and baked goods (which you will be avoiding anyway).
- **Corn:** Frequently genetically modified and can cause allergies in many people. Corn is also found in baking powder, caramel, dextrin, corn malt, cornstarch, and confectioners' sugar.
- **Beans:** Avoid because they contain saponins, which can be allergenic, and because their carbohydrate content is five times that of their protein content.

Enjoy the Best Protein Sources

During the detox diet we limit the amount of animal protein we eat each day, mostly because the animals have been fed things that we—and they—shouldn't be eating. We've already discussed how animals are exposed to harmful chemicals. Many are also raised on an unnatural diet. For example, lots of attention has been focused lately on chickens that are fed grains instead of their natural diet, which would include bugs and seeds. These grains increase the chickens' appetite and enhance their hormones so that they develop a larger muscle mass, which means they'll have more thigh and breast meat. What's more, many times these grains are treated with arsenic to keep rats away. This leaves us with unhealthy chickens and unhealthy eggs. Researchers have also determined that when chickens eat a high-grain diet, the fatty acid profile of their egg yolks becomes proinflammatory, with high levels of arachidonic acid rather than the anti-inflammatory omega-3 fatty acids eicosapentaenoic acid (EPA) and docosahexaenoic acid (DHA) that are prevalent when the chickens are fed their natural diet. Look for eggs that are marked "free range," which means that they are eating a natural diet. Not only are they healthier, but they taste better and they look a little bit different: the yolk has an orange tinge instead of a pure yellow color.

Just as we don't want to eat eggs that are high in arachidonic acid because of the chickens' unnatural diet, we also don't want to eat beef that's been grain fed and is high in arachidonic acid. People are always blaming beef for the rise in heart disease, but the fact is that cattle raised on a natural grass diet are just as rich in omega-3 fatty acids as fish but without the high levels of mercury. For more information, a great resource is the American Grassfed Association Web site (www.ameri cangrassfed.org).

Reducing Your Body Burden Through Better Nutrition

I've created very exact guidelines for what foods you can eat. Simply limiting your diet to these foods will make a huge impact on the amount of toxins and allergenic foods you're getting exposed to. What's more, these are the foods that have the highest nutrient content, which will help improve your health and allow for weight loss. You'll find more information about the foods you can eat in chapter 13, but here's a quick list:

- Locally grown, fresh organic fruits and vegetables (except for night-shade vegetables, as described above)
- Free-range chicken and turkey
- Grass-fed beef
- Wild-caught, low-mercury fish

While you're following the detox diet, you'll also be supplementing your nutrition with a detox shake. The shake is nutritionally sound, and the amino acids it contains help to detoxify your system. By avoiding the foods you are sensitive to, and introducing the shake for additional nutritional support, you enable your body to focus on detoxification, rather than fighting inflammation. The body heals best when it is at rest, and this 30-day plan allows your body to go on a healing vacation.

You won't be losing any nutrients by drinking the shake. Indeed, you'll be getting more nutrients than you're probably getting from standard American breakfast foods. It provides all the necessary vitamins and minerals while removing the toxins you were getting exposed to by eating processed and chemically enhanced foods.

Now that you have identified your symptoms, and have a better idea of what may be causing them, you're ready to start the program. The next section will teach you everything you need to know about how a good detoxification can help improve your health and how the specific health concerns you identified with the detox questionnaire may be caused by toxic exposure.

Part II
The Effect of Toxins on Health

Chapter 6
Good Health Begins with Clean Cells

Our body works like a garden. In a healthy environment, plants grow easily because they get sufficient sunlight and water, and the soil is rich with nutrients. Plants in a healthy garden will be resistant to infections and insects, will bloom with flowers and yield fruit. But even if there is adequate water and sun, when the soil is depleted of nutrients or contaminated with toxins or weeds, the garden will not be able to thrive. The plants will be more susceptible to infections, insects, and mold, and they may not be able to produce fruit.

We know that we have to tend a garden to grow the most beautiful and healthy plants. Well, the human body is very much the same. We must do everything we can to create a hospitable environment within our body, not only to survive, but to thrive. And we can't pick and choose among a variety of healthy lifestyle options: we must employ them all. We can exercise regularly and see a doctor once a year, but if we are exposed to toxins or eat a poor diet, our health will be adversely affected.

Good health begins on the smallest, cellular level. Our cells must have the resources they need to function and to repair and detoxify themselves. When our cells are deprived of necessary nutritional resources, or become toxic from accumulated chemicals and heavy metals, we lose our ability to heal ourselves in times of sickness and are unable to efficiently detoxify even when we are well. When this happens, the body begins to break down, leading to fatigue, weight gain, premature aging, susceptibility to illness, and more.

How Cells Work

Each cell is a microcosm of your overall self and a reflection of your health. In order to function, each and every cell requires the same things a person needs to survive: nutrients to create energy (proteins, fats, and carbohydrates) as well as oxygen and water.

The primary goal of every cell is to maintain homeostasis, or balance, while accomplishing its specific functions. Every cell is surrounded by a semipermeable fatty phospholipid membrane that separates it from other cells and from the external fluid environment. The cell membrane's most important function is to distinguish between the nutrients that should enter the cell and the toxins or chemicals that should not. The nutrients that cells can absorb include the carbohydrates, fat, and proteins that we have eaten, which have all been processed in the digestive tract. So when you are eating a diet that's healthful and has an adequate supply of protein, fat, and carbohydrates along with all the necessary vitamins, minerals, and cofactors, then your cells can carry out their functions correctly and remain healthy, which helps to keep the body healthy.

When healthy, this pliable cell membrane is comprised of the correct ratio of lipids and fatty acids. A diet that is deficient in healthy fats or has too many unhealthy transaturated fats will cause an imbalance and thereby make the cell membrane rigid, trapping toxins and waste products and causing cellular dysfunction. This situation can lead to diseases such as hardening of the arteries and high blood pressure. If you are also exposed to toxins such as mercury from tuna, pesticides from conventionally grown fruits and vegetables, or chemicals from industrial waste, these toxins can sneak through the cell membrane, contributing to poor health.

Cells Need Oxygen to Prevent Mitochondrial Dysfunction

Just like our body has organs with specific functions, our cells have organelles, or tiny structures, that carry out specific tasks. The organelles that create energy are called mitochondria. Mitochondria are also known as the powerhouses of the cell, because they convert carbohydrates into ATP (adenosine triphosphate), the fuel that keeps cells alive and helps to drive all other cellular processes.

Some cells have lots of mitochondria, literally tens of thousands, which are necessary if the cell has a great demand for energy, like the cells that make up the heart. Other cells, like skin cells or fat cells, don't operate as intensely and, needing much less ATP, have fewer mitochondria.

Under ordinary circumstances of aerobic metabolism, the oxygen in our system allows mitochondria to convert glucose into thirty-eight ATP molecules so that our cells can carry out their mission and energize our body. We have lots of energy, we can think clearly, we are able to easily maintain our weight, and our cells can properly detoxify themselves. However, if a cell is not getting enough oxygen the mitochondria need to produce energy through anaerobic metabolism (meaning without oxygen) and for each glucose molecule only two ATP molecules are produced, with lactic acid as the by-product.

Athletes are very familiar with the effects of anaerobic metabolism. When they are performing a high-intensity exercise like sprinting to first base, lunging to hit a tennis ball, or running up stairs, their bodies are rapidly trying to create energy to meet short-term energy needs. While this chemical process is inefficient, it gets the job done at an expense. The next day they may notice that their muscles are sore, and they may require a few days to recuperate. That soreness occurs because the muscles were using anaerobic metabolism to create fast energy, and the lactic acid formed in the muscles causes the cramps.

This situation is very similar to what happens when, over time, you are exposed to low-level toxins, chemicals, or heavy metals. Your cells become oxygen deprived or inefficient at creating ATP due to mitochondrial damage. That, in turn, forces your muscles to meet energy demands through anaerobic means, and lactic acid simultaneously accumulates in your muscles and tissues. But unlike the runner who experiences this over a short period of time (say, while running a sprint), a toxic body never reaches the end of the race. Inevitably, you begin to feel the symptoms of chronic muscle achiness and constant fatigue. This is one theory for why chronic fatigue syndrome and fibromyalgia syndrome occur.

EXERCISE REVERSES CELLULAR DYSFUNCTION

Exercise is really useful to help improve mitochondrial function because it stimulates the body to produce more mitochondria. Research published in the *European Journal of Applied Physiology* in 2009 showed that physical exercise increases mitochondrial function and reduces oxidative damage in skeletal muscle. However, the opposite is true as well: if we become sedentary our cells eventually lose mitochondrial function as they adapt to a stressless life situation.

The Weakest Link Theory

Cellular dysfunction affects each of us differently. It usually hits the weakest part of the body. That happens because the body tries to protect healthy, vital areas at the expense of less-vital areas. If you look at the results of your detox questionnaire, you can get a better understanding of where your weakest points are. The group of symptoms for which you scored the highest is likely associated with the area where your cells become dysfunctional first.

Doctors and researchers are just beginning to understand the science of mitochondrial dysfunction. Increased understanding will allow clinicians to address the roots of illness. More often than not, doctors address only the symptoms and not the cause. I believe that most symptoms are caused by, and clearly connected to, the health of your cells and how they are affected by toxins.

When Mitochondria Become Dysfunctional, Your Waistline Suffers

Mitochondria generate energy and control your metabolism by synthesizing oxygen with glucose that is produced from the foods you eat. The most important part of this three-step cycle is referred to as the "electron transport chain." In this stage, each glucose molecule shuttles electrons inside the mitochondrial membrane, combining with oxygen. The end result creates water and carbon dioxide, and generates your internal heat, or the energy you use to run your body and burn off calories.

This process is accomplished when you breathe clean air: you efficiently intake oxygen and release carbon dioxide. However, when oxygen is masked by other pollutants, or when the mitochondria are so dysfunctional that they cannot allow the oxygen to enter the cell membrane, the electron transport chain cannot function and the cell becomes inefficient. To understand this better, imagine what it would be like if your car only got two miles to the gallon instead of thirty-eight. You would need nineteen times the amount of gas to go the same distance. This is exactly why you may feel like you're always hungry, because in truth your tank is always empty. But when you keep eating, you interfere with your natural capacity to burn off these calories correctly, and they become stored for later use as body fat. The rub is, you never get around to using those calories, and it shows in your expanding waistline.

The Effects of Rapidly Aging AGEs

A second type of cellular catastrophe comes from eating a diet rich in refined sugar. Because that kind of diet lacks nutrients, it creates a toxic environment within our cells. What happens is that the sugar molecules we ingest attach to protein molecules in our cell membranes or even in our DNA. The new sugar-protein molecule is called an AGE (advanced glycation end product). These molecules interfere with normal metabolism, jam up the healing process, and, worst yet, have inflammatory and oxidative properties that literally age cells. Once an AGE is formed, it's irreversible: it sits inside cells, forming dysfunctional molecules, which in turn damage our cells even more.

The outward effect is wrinkles and sagging skin; the internal effect is cellular breakdown. AGEs have been linked to diabetes, cataract development, nerve damage, kidney disease, Alzheimer's disease, heart disease, and stroke.

AGEs are a disease of modern society. From the outside looking in, these toxic molecules are formed during cooking: that beautiful caramelized browning that occurs when you grill or broil or fry. We also produce AGEs when there's too much sugar in the bloodstream. Soft drinks, processed snacks, ice cream, candy, and other simple white carbs like pasta, white rice, and white potatoes all cause blood-sugar levels to swing rapidly back and forth, and when the sugar in our cells becomes too high for an extended period of time, AGEs develop.

However, the good news is that AGEs can be completely controlled by managing blood sugar and choosing different cooking methods. This is one of the most compelling reasons why the detox shake you will be drinking is so important: it limits your exposure to both of these kinds of food dilemmas. When you follow the 30-day program, you will be adhering to a diet of more complex carbohydrates, making you a lot less susceptible to forming AGEs.

SPECIAL SUPPLEMENTS TO REVERSE AGEs

The supplement benfotiamine is a synthetic fat-soluble derivative of vitamin B_1 that may help to reverse cells that have AGE formations. Also, the nutrients alpha-lipoic acid and quercetin are useful because they work as antioxidants that help prevent AGEs from forming.

The Effects of Oxidative Stress

Oxidation is a necessary part of turning sugar into ATP. To avoid becoming damaged during the process of combing sugar and oxygen, our cells have buffers, or antioxidants, that keep the oxidation reactions from getting out of control. However, if oxidation occurs in an uncontrolled fashion and antioxidants aren't around to do their job, damage occurs.

A good analogy is fire: When a fire is burning in a fireplace it can be easily controlled and will provide heat and light on a cold winter night. But if a fire is burning in the middle of your living room, it could burn down your whole house.

Toxic chemicals like mercury and lead increase cellular oxidation, as do nicotine, coffee, and simple sugars. When toxic exposures exceed the body's ability to detoxify itself, or if our antioxidant reserve is inadequate to neutralize it, oxidative stress occurs, leading to an uncontrolled fire burning in our cells. This can lead to cell damage and symptoms consistent with difficult-to-diagnose chronic syndromes like fibromyalgia, irritable bowel, and chronic fatigue syndromes.

By following the 30-day detox diet, you will be avoiding the foods and many of the chemicals that cause your cellular fire to burn out of

---

DIFFICULT DIAGNOSES

Fibromyalgia (FM) is usually classified as a soft tissue musculoskeletal condition. It causes intense, debilitating pain that can be constant and crippling. FM is often associated with another condition called chronic fatigue syndrome (CFS). Often symptoms related to FM or CFS are not consistent or not easily recognized or misdiagnosed. They can include fatigue, muscle achiness, difficulty concentrating, sore throat, recurrent infections, memory changes, and either weight gain or weight loss. I have found that these symptoms will often reverse or diminish once toxins that are putting oxidative stress on the cells are eliminated from the body.

control, causing oxidative stress, and instead nourish yourself with foods that are high in antioxidants, which will put you back in control of your cellular health.

The Problem with Free Radicals

As cells age, mitochondria are not able to replicate as efficiently. When fewer mitochondria are being produced, our cells become more susceptible to free radicals. Free radicals are unstable atoms that attack other molecules in order to gain stability and may damage cellular components in the process. Some free radicals are produced in our cells, while others are produced from chemicals, toxins, infections, and even inflammatory foods that we consume. However, all free radicals add to the oxidative stress that is a by-product of our day-to-day lives and are directly linked to illness.

Our cells need sufficient antioxidants to bind up and buffer free radicals. The body produces three types of antioxidants on its own: superoxide dismutase, catalase, and glutathione peroxidase. However, if our cells are not functioning properly and we cannot make these antioxidants, we need to increase our antioxidants through diet. In order to aid our cellular defenses, we want to both reduce the amount of toxic foods and chemicals we get exposed to and focus on eating foods that are high in antioxidants, like fresh fruits and vegetables.

Cells Need Water

Next to oxygen, water is probably the most important nutrient for the health of our cells. There is water both inside and surrounding cells, and it is used to transport nutrients, vitamins, and minerals. A proper balance of minerals is required both within cells and in their surrounding environment, but these minerals must be dissolved in water to be transported properly. Increasing your water intake to about one to two liters (about half a gallon) daily allows you to become properly hydrated and thereby bring more fluid into cells to literally flush out toxins.

Cells are constantly absorbing nutrients and toxins, and getting rid of waste through the fluid-filled space between them called interstitial fluid. The interstitial fluid is composed of water, minerals, electrolytes, proteins, and toxins. When cells attempt to pump toxins into the interstitial fluid, you may experience fluid retention or swelling in your hands, feet, or face. When fluid retention occurs from lymph stuck in the tissue, this is called lymph edema, and its hallmark is that the skin does not indent when compressed. For example, if you push your finger into an ankle swollen from lymph edema, no indentation remains when you remove your finger. If the swelling is just from fluid retention, your finger's indent will remain, like the lines you see on your ankle when you remove your socks at the end of the day.

Interstitial fluid filters into the lymphatic system, circulates through your blood on the way to the liver, and eventually exits through the colon. If the water you consume does not have the right amount of minerals like calcium and magnesium, as well as electrolytes like sodium, potassium, and chloride, the entire process is thrown off. In addition, if your drinking water is heavily chlorinated or contains insecticides, pesticides, or heavy metals, then you are inadvertently delivering those chemicals directly to the cells. In chapter 3 we discussed the best ways to make sure that you are drinking clean, mineral-rich water.

If you are constantly hot or drawn to drinking cold water, that's a clear sign that your body is not functioning properly. It also is a sign that your cells are not functioning properly. When you are hot, your cells are not using energy efficiently, and you're not making ATP properly. When you're producing energy efficiently, you're not producing an excess amount of heat.

Detoxification Resolves Cellular Dysfunction

Our cells need to maintain a state of balance, or homeostasis, by protecting the cell membrane, which in turn helps to maintain mitochondrial function and the important processes of our body. Therefore our goal is to find ways to restore our balance on the cellular level. That's exactly what a good detoxification does. It removes harmful toxins from the system and makes simple, positive dietary modifications to add more healthful nutrients. By making informed choices about the foods you eat, and how you prepare them, you are well on your way to beginning your detox.

Keeping Cells Healthy Is Your Job

Most traditional doctors are not thinking about your health on a cellular level. It is just not what they are trained to do. A doctor's mission is to look at the big picture of your health and to try to come up with treatments for your current symptoms that will improve the overall picture.

My goal is to get you to look at medicine in an entirely new light. Instead of a symptom-disease-treatment approach, my practice informs patients about prevention as well as treatment. Now that you understand how important it is to keep your cells healthy, you can begin to take control of your own health and be responsible for your health care so that illness does not become part of your future. And if you are experiencing symptoms now, you can fully understand their underlying cause with the goal of acting proactively to treat it.

Not every health problem will come down to cellular health or be rooted in toxic exposure. A person with chronic fatigue or fibromyalgia could be tired or achy because of diabetes, heart disease, or cancer, and these conditions all need to be investigated. But when those diseases are ruled out, we need to figure out what the real cause is. And that's where it's important to focus on issues that are less commonly addressed in conventional medicine.

In the next few chapters you will find more about how toxins specifically affect your health and how the detox can help reverse symptoms you may be having by potentially addressing their underlying cause.

Chapter 7
Clear Your Mind for Better Thinking

The brain oversees and monitors all aspects of proper body function, including detoxification. Your unique combination of brain chemicals, called neurotransmitters, influences how you think, feel, and behave. These neurotransmitters are generally divided into excitatory (activating) or inhibitory (calming) groups. The excitatory neurotransmitters include dopamine, norepinephrine, and epinephrine. The inhibitory neurotransmitters include serotonin and GABA. If your neurotransmitters are out of balance and you have, for example, too much dopamine and not enough serotonin that would make you susceptible to anxiety because you have too much excitatory dopamine stimulation and also susceptible to depression because you have too little serotonin.

Neurotransmitters remain in balance along with your overall health. And toxins can affect brain chemistry just like they affect your other internal systems, changing the way we think and feel, and even how much energy we have. These pollutants can either directly poison brain cells or cause inflammation of the brain. This chapter will explore what happens when the brain is affected by a toxic environment, whether external or internally created.

The symptoms and conditions listed below do not occur in a vacuum:

like other aspects of your health they all stem from one cause or another. Neurological symptoms can be directly linked to stressful life events, specific illnesses, and even medications. If you've already been diagnosed with a neurological ailment, such as anxiety, depression, attention deficit disorder (ADD), or even dementia, and your symptoms have not resolved themselves with time, medication, psychological counseling, or other types of therapy, your mental health may be affected by your environment.

For example, brain fog or forgetfulness is a common complaint; one that is often associated with aging. However, losing your attention or becoming more forgetful is not necessarily "normal." Instead, it's a clear symptom that the brain is not functioning properly and may have become toxic. The goal of detoxification is to identify what is causing your brain symptoms so that you can think clearly well into your old age. The good news is that when you complete a thorough detoxification, you may find that your thinking quickly improves.

A toxic brain can also manifest as fatigue, irritability, or mood swings. These emotional symptoms could be linked to neurological manifestations of hormone imbalances, such as when women go through menopause or men experience andropause (male menopause). In such cases people can develop anxiety and depression or find they have difficulty making decisions or staying energetic. Luckily, if and when you follow the detox, you will find that it's easier to handle whatever stresses you have, regardless of the source of your anxiety.

In the first section of the book, we discussed how toxins like heavy metals, pesticides, and insecticides interfere with the central nervous system's ability to function properly. These toxins can also directly poison the ability of brain cells to produce and recognize neurotransmitters. While most of us are not likely to become exposed to very large concentrations of toxins, which would cause an obvious and immediate reaction that would send us to the emergency room, we are all getting exposed to small amounts of these same chemicals, and over time they can potentially interfere with the brain's ability to function.

At the same time, inflammatory food reactions are also toxic to the brain and can cause neurological symptoms. Usually, we think of food allergies as immediately causing rashes, hives, or even severe swelling of the airway that can become life threatening. However, the delayed type of food sensitivity can cause brain symptoms similar to those seen with other toxic exposures, including fatigue, brain fog, difficulty concentrating, irritability, and mood changes.

I have seen significant improvement in many of the neurological symptoms listed below after my patients followed the detox diet for as few as thirty days. I have also witnessed the return of symptoms when the culprit-foods were reintroduced.

It is interesting to note that neurological symptoms from chronic low-level toxin exposure or food intolerance can cause stimulation, depression, or both stimulation and depression of the nervous system at the same time. Again, there is not a great deal of research on this topic; however, in my opinion this occurs because every patient has a different capacity for and method of handling their toxic load. As a consequence, some people may develop irritability, anxiety, and insomnia from chronic exposures, while others will experience depression and fatigue. It is like the way some people become energized after one glass of alcohol, while others become sleepy. Similarly, when someone who is sensitive to wheat or sugar eats doughnuts or even a muffin for breakfast they may feel temporarily energized from the sugar high, while others may develop fatigue, extreme sleepiness, or difficulty concentrating.

Toxins Poison the Brain and Central Nervous System

Under ordinary circumstances, the brain works like the command center of a military operation, sending cellular signals from the central nervous system (CNS) to the peripheral nervous system (PNS), which instructs the body to make sure the organs, hormones, and other processes are working together to maintain balance. The CNS, or headquarters, is separated from direct contact with the rest of the body by the blood-brain barrier, which selectively prevents chemicals, toxins, and proteins from entering and disturbing brain function.

However, when the brain is poisoned by being overwhelmed with toxic chemicals, inflammatory foods, or even infections, the body responds by creating an immune system response that supersedes the brain's control mechanisms. Inflammatory chemicals and immune cells are released either at the sight of an infection or throughout the entire body in an attempt to isolate and remove the offending and irritating chemicals and toxins. This is not unlike what happens after a terrorist attack, when military police heighten their level of surveillance and scrutiny of all potentially threatening occurrences. And just as a sudden, powerful military response is never completely precise and efficient in its execution, our immune response can also cause collateral damage. For example, the blood-brain barrier can become compromised because of inflammation, allowing chemicals to enter and irritate the brain. The autonomic nervous system, which typically functions to maintain order through the PNS, gets shut down in favor of the sympathetic nervous system, which operates during times of fight or flight. And if your body's response is overly aggressive or occurs for an extended period of time—because it has been exposed to toxins or inflammatory foods for an extended period—then the damage can be devastating to your brain and body.

Toxins that affect the brain include low levels of pesticide exposure. An interesting 2006 study conducted by the Harvard School of Public Health and published in the *Annals of Neurology* showed that individuals reporting exposure to pesticides had a 70 percent higher incidence of Parkinson's disease than those not reporting exposure. I believe that pesticide accumulation over time causes poisoning of the brain's dopamine receptors. Hopefully, by following the guidelines in this book you can limit your exposure and decrease your susceptibility to neurodegenerative conditions.

Heavy metals like mercury and lead are toxins that both directly poison cells in the brain and can cause an inappropriate autoimmune response that affects brain function. If you are exposed to heavy metals, your body's first objective is to bind the toxins so that they can be removed. A group of proteins called metallothionein is solely responsible for this purpose. However, if your exposure to heavy metals is too great for metallothionein to manage, the heavy metals get shuttled to the body's storage areas, or fat cells. If you do not have enough fat, then the heavy metals will accumulate in other cells throughout the body or brain. The level of accumulation eventually affects the cells' ability to conduct normal functions, just like your work efficiency will eventually decline from having a cluttered desk.

We know from past history that people exposed to mercury while producing felt for hats developed Mad Hatter syndrome: a complex of mercury-related symptoms that includes inflammation of the mouth, diarrhea, loss of muscular movement, tremors, sensorineural impairment, and emotional instability. This group of symptoms is a perfect example of how mercury can be directly toxic to the brain and central nervous system function. The afflicted individuals were known to have worked with mercury, its levels were excessively high in their blood, and the symptoms disappeared when they were no longer exposed to it. But mercury can cause permanent damage, so unfortunately some of the workers were never fully functional again.

Mercury and lead can also have a devastating effect on the developing brains of children. A 2005 article in *Environmental Health Perspectives* found in national blood-mercury-prevalence data from the Centers for Disease Control and Prevention (CDC) that between three hundred thousand and six hundred thousand newborn children each year have umbilical cord blood mercury at a level associated with loss of IQ. More recently, research from a 2008 study published in the same journal showed that children's intellectual functioning at six years of age was impaired by blood-lead concentrations well below the current CDC definition of elevated blood lead, which is 10 mcg/dl. The study suggested that some type of intervention should be made if a child's blood-lead level is above 5 mcg/dl.

Children can develop brain dysfunction from indirect and low-level exposure to lead and mercury. The exposure to mercury seems to mostly come from excessive fish consumption, beginning during fetal development from the pregnant mother's diet. Pregnant mothers should not have mercury fillings placed or removed because the mercury that is released can be transferred to the fetus. In addition, children are still frequently exposed to lead in old paint, contaminated water, and even dishware with lead glaze.

Inflammation in the Brain

Heavy metals cause inflammation in the central nervous system that's separate from the effects of other toxins. Mercury, in particular, has a very profound impact on the immune system. The FDA reports on its Web site that some individuals have an allergy or sensitivity to mercury in silver dental fillings, which can cause oral lesions or other contact reactions. In addition, the immune response from mercury can lead to inflammation, neurotoxicity, and neurodegeneration, which result in memory changes, mental confusion, and possibly dementia.

Inflammation caused by an immune response can affect your neurological functions. As we discussed earlier in this chapter, the immune response can cause collateral damage: affecting neuron cell integrity, brain cells' ability to heal themselves and properly produce neurotransmitters and antioxidants, and eventually compromising the blood-brain barrier. Sometimes the immune response is just too great and, as a result, our brain cells get affected. They get caught in the crossfire of the war between our immune response and the foreign agents, and unfortunately become collateral damage. This is similar to the way chemotherapy can adversely affect brain cells: ideally it is supposed to kill only cancer cells, but it almost invariably affects every other cell in the body as well.

The problem with inflammation is that in order for it to resolve, the initial cause of the inflammation must be identified and removed.

Otherwise the body will continue to have an out-of-control immune response. Once the cause of the problem is determined and removed, the immune system will quickly return to a normal level of function and regulation. With our detox diet, we hope to simplify as much as possible the process of recognizing and removing irritants, so the body can function at a normal level and get back to doing only what it's supposed to do.

When inflammation affects the brain, we can't produce enough neurotransmitters. These are the chemical messengers that govern the proper workings of the brain. Without the right amounts of neurotransmitters, you'll feel out of sorts both physically and mentally. However, when you lower inflammation in the brain through detox, you help rebalance your brain chemistry so that you are better able to handle whatever stresses you have in your life.

For example, if you are currently taking medicine to control depression or anxiety, both of which are signs of neurotransmitter imbalances in the brain, you may be able to wean yourself off this type of medication after a thorough detoxification. Of course, you can't just stop taking this type of medication without the supervision of your doctor. Antidepressants and anti-anxiety medications can become habit forming: your brain becomes dependent on them, so they must be decreased gradually. However, many of my patients find that, with time, they are able to wean themselves from those prescriptions and stay off them.

Alex Reversed Memory Loss

Alex was a successful psychoanalyst for many years. Yet he found himself having a great deal of difficulty remembering his patients' names and their stories. He came to me to help him resolve his memory and attention problems. Even though he changed his diet and completed the detox, Alex's symptoms had not improved. After working together for about three years, we finally discovered that his symptoms might be coming from mercury. We did an appropriate mercury detoxification, which included eliminating fish from his diet and, finally, removing his old mercury fillings. Alex was astonished that his memory and quality of life were transformed within weeks of going through this thorough heavy metal detoxification process. If the symptoms were only caused by his diet, they should have improved after he began avoiding fish and going through a detox. However, it was not until he had his silver (mercury) fillings removed that he noticed the biggest difference in his memory. This demonstrated to me that his symptoms were from sensitivity to the fillings and not just from dietary toxicity.

Even though it was necessary for Alex to have his fillings removed, not everyone needs to go through this tedious process. But if your mercury-related symptoms remain after completing the 30-day detox diet, you may want to consider this option. Removing a toxic irritant from your body is like removing a stone from your shoe. The goal is to find the stone. For Alex, it was the mercury fillings.

Infections in the Body Affect the Brain

Certain infections like Lyme disease, bartonella, babesia, and ehrlichiosis, all of which can be contracted from a tick bite, as well as molds like stachybotrys, penicillium, and even candida can produce toxins that affect the central nervous system. Unfortunately, the majority of people who get a tick bite or are exposed to mold never know it. The ticks that carry these infections can be found in all fifty states and in Canada, but they are very small and are excellent at camouflaging themselves on the human body. One of the telltale signs of a tick bite is a bull's-eye rash at the site of the bite; however, this only occurs 50 percent of the time. Symptoms of a generalized infection related to the tick bite can develop, including achy muscles and achy joints.

If you are lucky enough to identify the signs of a tick bite, then appropriate blood tests for tick infections and treatment with antibiotics can be started immediately. However, if you never see the tick bite or rash and your symptoms are not recognized early, the infection can develop into a chronic form that agitates your immune system and produces low levels of toxins that affect your CNS. If you have had symptoms of achy muscles, achy joints, and now are experiencing fatigue, light or sound sensitivity, or brain fog, it is worth talking with your doctor about testing for these infections and, if present, treating them appropriately.

Molds can cause another class of infections and brain irritation and yet are easily overlooked as a cause of chronic brain symptoms. This is because mold can live under carpets, in ventilation shafts, or behind walls, so you may never even see the telltale signs of mold growth that would make you suspicious of their presence. Symptoms of mold toxicity include fatigue, achy muscles, achy joints, mental confusion, and brain fog. If you have these symptoms and no other cause has been discovered, you may want to thoroughly evaluate your home for mold, as we discussed in chapter 4. If you have mold in your home, take your findings to your doctor so you can decide if you need additional allergy testing to clarify which mold is the problem. Once it is identified, it must be completely remediated in order to improve your symptoms.

As you go through the detox process, you may find that your symptoms of brain toxicity improve. This may be because you are better able to manage the toxins you are exposed to or because your immune system is becoming better balanced. It has been very interesting for me to see in my practice that two patients with the same type of tick-borne infections can have completely different symptoms. Some of my colleagues and I even speculate that there are a great deal more patients with Lyme disease than what we know about, but who never complain of any symptoms because their immune systems are somehow keeping the infection from progressing. But we end up seeing these patients after their immune systems become weak from developing a different infection, another tick bite, or even getting exposed to molds. Once the immune system gets overburdened, the Lyme disease becomes active and symptoms occur. That's why the detox diet is so powerful: it quickly helps to eliminate many potential causes of exposure that can upset the immune response. And even though it's not going to get rid of all of the potential causes, it might get rid of enough to allow the body to either begin to heal itself or start to function properly on its own.

Foods Affect Thinking and Feeling

Food cravings can be a clear sign of brain toxicity caused by poor internal health or dietary choices. Cravings for sugar or sweets might indicate that your digestive tract is off balance: that you are producing too much yeast, which can be caused by taking excessive antibiotics or steroids, drinking chlorinated water, or stress. Once yeast gets out of balance, you may start having mental health problems like brain fog.

Excessive yeast growth causes us to crave even more sugar because yeast requires sugar to survive. That's part of why you may feel groggy after eating too many sweets: the yeast in the digestive tract is converting sugar into alcohol and all of a sudden you've become a human microbrewery.

The detox diet helps to selectively starve certain types of yeast because you will not be eating the yeast's main food source: excessive amounts of sugar. You'll find that your food cravings end as well as your mood swings.

Not only does the digestive tract house most of the immune system, there are also more serotonin receptors in the digestive tract than are in the brain. In fact, the digestive tract is sometimes referred to as the body's second brain. That's in part why we feel satisfied or relieved after we eat a piece of chocolate or a sweet. The chocolate message isn't immediately sent to the brain; neurotransmitter-like chemicals in the chocolate stimulate serotonin receptors right in the digestive tract.

This feeling of satisfaction can be quickly followed by feeling shaky, jittery, or tired: your blood sugar is dropping after the spike that occurs when you eat sweets like cakes or cookies or simple carbs like pasta. Then you begin to produce insulin that takes all that sugar out of the blood and drives it into the cells, but because it's responding to such a high sugar spike the body overproduces insulin, and then our blood sugar crashes again. When your blood sugar goes low, you produce adrenaline and another hormone, glucagon, to try to stimulate either your own production of sugar to balance the low blood sugar, which leaves you feeling anxious and irritable. The goal of the detox diet is to stabilize your blood sugar and take you off this roller coaster ride.

Other foods, like those we discussed in chapter 5, can also cause inflammation that affects the central nervous system. A good example is the story of Thomas, whose gluten sensitivity caused him to have severe neurological problems. Once he completed the detox diet, his schizophrenia resolved very quickly, and he was able to go back to work.

Now that you have a good idea about how your brain works and how toxins affect your thinking, let's take a closer look at how toxins affect the rest of the body, starting with the immune system.

Chapter 8
Reduce Inflammation and Improve Immune Function

The human body was not designed to handle an ever-increasing toxic load. Once your capacity is reached, your body may begin to unnaturally recognize itself as a "foreign" problem, in much the same way that it reacts to allergic substances, bacteria, or infections. The immune system triggers a switch that can cause your body to start attacking itself, leading to a group of conditions known as autoimmune disease.

Autoimmune diseases include rheumatoid arthritis, systemic lupus, Crohn's disease, and even asthma. The principle common to these conditions is that they involve the body inappropriately attacking its own cells. No one knows for sure why the body's immune system mistakes its own cells for foreign intruders and thus attacks itself, but some suspect one or more of the following:

- **Genetic susceptibility:** An increased risk of developing a disease based on your family's medical history. This often occurs in patients with type 2 diabetes as well as in patients with immune-related diseases including allergies and asthma.
- **Molecular mimicry:** This occurs when the immune system correctly recognizes and attacks an infection but the antibodies it

produces also attack healthy cells that have a similar molecular structure to the infection, such as cartilage cells found in the joints. When this occurs, the antibodies negatively affect the joints, causing inflammation. This often occurs in cases of rheumatoid arthritis or ankylosing spondylitis.

- **The hygiene hypothesis:** It is speculated that lack of early childhood exposure to infectious agents, good bacteria, and parasites may increase susceptibility to allergies and autoimmune disease. This theory is often used to explain the increase in allergies and autoimmune diseases since industrialization in more developed countries. The use of antibacterial soap, pesticides, and chlorinated water has sterilized the environment, which may lead to an imbalanced immune response.
- **Heavy metal toxicity:** Mercury and cadmium are two heavy metals that can provoke an autoimmune response.

Inflammation as an Immune Response

The first symptoms of any immune response include inflammation, pain, and swelling. These symptoms are your body's way of telling you that you have sensitivity to something, and they can be very useful: when you have a sore throat, that's your signal to see a health care provider to make sure you don't have an infection like pharyngitis or strep throat. However, if you find that you get a sore throat every time you eat a particular food or are exposed to something in your environment, and that sore throat never turns out to be an infection, then you may want to consider removing the offending toxin and seeing if that helps alleviate your symptoms.

The area in your body where inflammation develops determines your particular set of symptoms. This area I call your weak spot. Just as we each have certain strengths and weaknesses in life, each of our bodies is unique and slightly flawed. Some people may find that they are very good at running but have poor hand-eye coordination. Some people never seem to get sick, but when they do, they always get strep throat. Some people may find that they always get urinary tract infections. The part of the body that develops symptoms first is the weak spot. In the case of an immune response, the first sign of sickness will be in your weak spot because it will be the first area to develop inflammation. For example, if you have seasonal allergies you may find that in the spring your symptoms are concentrated in the nose and eyes, while other people with the same allergies are hit with coughing or wheezing.

The detox diet prescribed in this book is a very general treatment strategy in that it helps with a lot of body functions all at once. However, you can fine-tune your protocol based on your weak spot by incorporating the right nutritional supplements, listed in Appendix I. If your symptoms are severe and you find that they have not resolved or improved by at least 50 percent after completing the 30-day plan, or if you feel after the first week that your symptoms are worsening, then you should immediately see your health care provider to determine if you have a medical problem that may need to be treated with prescription medications to bring the symptoms under control. While on the prescription medications, it is still safe to continue the meal plan with the goal of reducing your need for the medications later.

WHAT'S YOUR WEAK SPOT?

You can easily determine your weak spot by looking at your scores on the detox questionnaire. The categories that have the highest scores are your weakest points. Then your job is to address your weakest areas by discovering what is causing your symptoms. After that, you will be able to reinforce those areas to help improve your health now and for the long run.

Diseases Related to Inflammation

In medicine, many of the diseases that involve inflammation end with "itis." A wide range of conditions and diseases are linked with acute and chronic inflammation or have an inflammatory component:

- acid reflux/heartburn
- acne
- allergies and sensitivities
- Alzheimer's disease
- asthma
- atherosclerosis
- bronchitis
- cancer
- carditis
- celiac disease
- chronic pain
- cirrhosis
- colitis
- Crohn's disease
- dementia
- dermatitis
- diabetes
- dry eyes
- eczema
- edema
- emphysema
- fibromyalgia
- gastroenteritis
- gingivitis
- heart disease
- hepatitis
- high blood pressure
- insulin resistance
- interstitial cystitis
- joint pain/arthritis/ rheumatoid arthritis
- metabolic syndrome (syndrome X)
- myositis
- nephritis
- obesity
- osteopenia
- osteoporosis
- Parkinson's disease
- periodontal disease
- polyarteritis nodosa
- polychondritis
- psoriasis
- scleroderma
- sinusitis
- Sjögren's syndrome
- spastic colon
- systemic candidiasis
- tendonitis
- urinary tract infections
- vaginitis (a vaginal irritation or inflammation stemming from yeast or bacterial infection)

The Switch Phenomenon

Early stages of inflammation and autoimmune issues might include rashes on the skin (eczema), chronic sinus infections, allergies, asthma, joint stiffness, or ongoing digestive problems. Often these symptoms occur for long periods of time and if they are bothersome enough are usually treated with prescription medications aimed at controlling symptoms. During this treatment period, there can be times when the symptoms appear to become less severe or even stop occurring, only to be followed by a shift to some other set of more severe symptoms. This is often referred to as the "switch phenomenon."

A perfect example of this is when a child develops a rash and is diagnosed with atopic dermatitis. The mother is told to try removing dairy products from the diet, and the rash clears. As a teenager, the same child is told to eat more dairy products in order to build strong bones, but this time, rather that developing a rash, she develops a chronic sinus or throat infection. If the dairy products are removed, the symptoms go away. However, because it is thought to be "difficult" to avoid dairy products altogether, they are not completely removed from the diet and the symptoms work themselves further into the body; eventually asthma develops.

And if these kinds of symptoms are continually suppressed, for example with antibiotics to control sinus infections, antihistamines to control sinus congestion, and finally steroid medications to control asthma, and the cause of the symptoms is not removed, then at some point the symptoms will affect a completely different part of the body, in a process that is gradually spiraling out of control and that could at some point switch into becoming a more serious autoimmune disease.

Because inflammation can occur anywhere in the body, the switch phenomenon occurs quite often without our knowledge. For example, a patient may have sinusitis that can be cleared by prescription medication, but if the underlying cause has not been determined, the same patient may at some later point begin to develop joint stiffness and, eventually, arthritis. Chronic digestive cramping and inflammation (colitis) symptoms may clear, only for the same patient later to develop bladder inflammation (cystitis). Many times you may find yourself running back to the doctor to get another medication to treat what is thought to be another infection or to simply suppress the symptoms of inflammation. When symptoms are recurrent and do not resolve, it is a very good time to try detoxification.

If you had a stone in your shoe, you would take it out of the shoe to remove the irritation to your foot. If you decided to leave the stone in your shoe because you are just too busy to remove it, you might temporarily adjust to the pain, but at the end of the day you're going to have a sore foot. The longer you leave the stone in, the more irritated your foot will become, and you may even develop a callus if you leave it in long enough. Well, why not just stop and take out that stone so your foot will feel better? Why not just remove the cause of your symptoms before your symptoms become a big problem? That's what a good detoxification is all about.

In the case of inflammation, you will learn that many causes can be environmentally related. If the cause of your symptoms is identified and then avoided, there is a very good chance that your symptoms will stabilize and the illness can be reversed. By avoiding the most likely food allergies and doing your best to eat organically grown foods that are free of pesticides, you may find, within a month or sooner, that your symptoms begin to improve. In my practice I find that with diet modification alone, patients can have as much as a 50 percent improvement in their symptoms after following the detox diet. Of course everyone is different, but the good news is that it will not hurt you to make this type of modification in your life.

Best of all, if the symptoms are brought under control, and the offending agent is never reintroduced, there is a very good chance that autoimmune disease will not become a part of your life, even in patients with a family history of autoimmune disease.

Symptoms of Failed Immune Function

The symptoms of inflammation below are grouped into the body areas affected. Many symptoms can be attributed to some type of immune system response. However, to keep things simple remember that all are ultimately linked to inflammation.

Head

dizziness

faintness

headaches

Eyes

bags or dark circles under the eyes

blurred or tunnel vision

swollen, reddened, or sticky eyelids

watery or itchy eyes

Ears

drainage from ear

earaches, ear infections

itchy ears

Nose

excessive mucus

hay fever

sinus problems

sneezing attacks

stuffy nose

Mouth/Throat

canker sores

chronic coughing

gagging, frequent need to clear throat

sore throat, hoarseness, loss of voice

swollen or discolored tongue, gums, lips

Skin

acne

excessive sweating

flushing

hair loss

hives, rashes, dry skin

Lungs

asthma

bronchitis

chest congestion

difficulty breathing

shortness of breath

Joints/Muscle

arthritis

feeling of weakness or tiredness

pain or aches in joints

pain or aches in muscles

stiffness or limitation of movement

Allergies

Many people have developed allergies to a wide range of substances and at a rate that seems to escalate every year. There are many theories as to why allergies occur. As mentioned, some scientists and doctors believe in the hygiene hypothesis: that allergy is more prevalent because of a lack of early childhood exposure to microorganisms that are necessary to modulate the immune system. The mechanism of action is thought to be triggered by an imbalance in the white-blood-cell-mediated immune response that stems from having developed in a sterilized environment during the first months of life. Because of this, the immune system does not develop in a way that it can handle toxins, certain foods, or environmental exposures like pollen, plants, or mold in the same way it would have if there had been more germs for it to combat early in its development.

Others believe that infants who are fed formula instead of breast milk may be more susceptible to allergies because they are not receiving the right antibodies from their mothers. Still others link the increased risk in developing allergies to overexposure to certain allergens or to pollutants, or to a decrease in the body's capacity to manage the body burden.

How Allergies Affect Overall Health

Once an allergy has developed, you typically remain sensitive to that particular substance for your entire life, even if you don't have symptoms. For example, you may have had allergies as a kid, but during your twenties and thirties your symptoms seemed to go away. Usually, that doesn't mean that you are no longer allergic but that the switch phenomenon has occurred or your body burden has in some way reduced itself.

Your symptoms will resolve themselves when you take stress off the immune system. For example, if you have pollen allergies and usually experience associated symptoms in the spring, you are less likely to have symptoms if you are able to avoid other toxins that might be contributing to your body burden. Your barrel is less full, so to speak, and you can stay below the threshold where your body will react. So even though you will continue to have an immune response when you come in contact with pollen, if you avoid other things that trigger an immune response it will make it less likely that you will have an allergic reaction. Many of my patients are amazed to find that after following the 30-day detox diet they have fewer or no seasonal allergy symptoms and don't need their allergy medications any longer.

Food allergies can trigger responses that are similar to those from environmental exposures. In controlled studies many foods and additives have been implicated in cases of chronic rhinitis, bronchial asthma, atopic eczema, and migraine headaches. As we discussed in the previous chapter, many of my patients with long-standing mental symptoms, including ADD and ADHD, who have not been helped by many years of conventional medical treatment, have experienced rapid relief of their symptoms when they have avoided certain foods.

A study published in the *Lancet* in 1978, and frequently referenced, shows that some foods cause a wide spectrum of disabling symptoms in people who are sensitive to them. The authors stated that a prominent difference between conventional allergic reactions, such as skin rash, and food sensitivities is that the patient is usually unaware of the link between the culprit-food and the reaction they are having. They may even be unaware that the symptom is related to food sensitivity, especially if the agent is a favorite food eaten on a daily basis or a food they often eat in large quantities. The foods most frequently implicated, from most common to least common, include wheat (78 percent of reported cases), oranges (65 percent), eggs (45 percent), milk (37 percent), and sugar (33 percent).

Again, in the detox diet the foods that are most likely to cause symptoms are completely eliminated for thirty days, and then reintroduced one at a time. If symptoms reoccur when a food is reintroduced, it is a sure sign that sensitivity to that food is present. Time and again I've seen my patients experience far fewer reactions or consistently milder reactions when they reintroduce wheat, sugar, dairy products, and soy after eliminating them on the detox diet, because their total body burden has been reduced.

Remember, a toxin is any substance that causes an adverse reaction in the body. Even though we usually think of chemicals and heavy metals as toxins, because a very small exposure can cause a very significant adverse reaction in the body, foods can also be considered toxins if they trigger an immune response. Specific foods can create inflammation in the body, which can cause the kinds of symptoms we've discussed, but inflammation can also cause swelling in the lymphatic system and tissue of the body, which prevents proper drainage and detoxification of our cells. If the offending food is not avoided, the chronic inflammation will cause toxins to build up, which will eventually lead to cellular dysfunction, organ dysfunction, and potentially even chronic disease. So by identifying and avoiding the food or chemical that's causing inflammation in your body, you have a chance to prevent the progression of your symptoms and potentially reverse illness.

Steve Reversed Joint Pain by Changing His Diet

Steve was a personal trainer who came to see me regarding his joint and muscle stiffness. He told me that his previous doctor had diagnosed him with degenerative osteoarthritis, even though he was only fifty years old. His joint stiffness affected his hips, knees, lower spine, hands, and thumbs, and the symptoms were constant during the day. He had tried many different types of anti-inflammatory medications, and the most effective ones only provided temporary improvement.

After a thorough checkup and completing the detox questionnaire, we realized that Steve was otherwise in an excellent state of health. He trained regularly at a nationally renowned gym, and his diet was relatively clean. On his first visit he scored a 28 overall on the detox questionnaire. Because he didn't have any other symptoms, we decided to do blood tests to check for markers of immune system dysfunction or nutritional deficiencies and to start him on the detox diet.

Steve finished the first 30-day program without complaint. When he came in to be retested, we found that his joint symptoms were 50 percent better. He reported that he felt like he had more energy, was less moody, had less abdominal gas and bloating, that his seasonal allergies were improved, and that he had better urinary flow. His questionnaire score went from 28 to 13.

However, Steve was leery about reintroducing foods that might cause inflammation, so he decided to stay with the program for another thirty days. After the second month, he found that he felt another 50 percent better. He had improved stamina and more range of motion in his joints. He began to add foods back into his daily routine. Steve found that dairy products caused mucus formation in his sinuses and throat. When he added certain spices, they caused him to get more digestive gas. And when he reintroduced the nightshade vegetables, his joint stiffness returned.

Steve continues to follow a modified version of the 30-day detox so that his symptoms are contained. He knows which foods he can eat and which he can't. By avoiding foods that cause inflammation, he helps his whole body feels better.

Infections and Inflammation

Another type of environmental exposure that causes inflammation is infection. The types of infections most closely associated with inflammation of the joints, connective tissues, and central nervous system and that potentially contribute to the symptoms listed earlier come from tick bites. These include Lyme disease (borrelia), babesia, bartonella, and ehrlichiosis. If you are able to get appropriate antibiotic treatment early, these infections will cure quickly. However, many people who get tick bites do not see an immediate onset of symptoms and therefore do not seek treatment right away. Instead, they experience a slow progression of worsening health, increased fatigue, joint stiffness, memory changes, and even fevers and chills that can sometimes go misdiagnosed for months or years.

The reason these infections, and in particular Lyme disease, are so difficult to detect is because they produce certain toxins that affect our immune system's response and our nervous system's perception of the infection. These toxins are created to allow the infection a way to avoid immune system detection and thereby improve their ability to reproduce, until they get to a critical threshold point where you start experiencing symptoms. These toxins then not only affect your immediate health but affect your body's ability to detoxify itself.

Remember, if you find that after completing the 30-day detox diet your symptoms of inflammation have not improved, please see your health care provider and ask them to consider an infection from a tick bite as part of their differential diagnosis, and make sure they do appropriate blood work.

Inflammation of Joints and Muscles

Inflammation in the muscles and joints is often caused by foods, including nightshade vegetables like tomatoes, white potatoes, eggplants, and peppers. These contain saponins, which are chemicals the plant produces to help protect itself from microbial and insect attack. However, saponins can cause inflammation in some susceptible individuals. Once you are done with the initial 30-day detox diet, you may want to reintroduce this group of fruits and vegetables; however, if you get symptoms from eating them, please listen to your body and keep them out of your diet.

Even osteoarthritis, considered a degenerative joint condition in which joints become worn over time, is believed to have a relationship to inflammation. Not everybody gets osteoarthritis as they get older, but certainly if a person has inflammation in their body, they're more susceptible to prematurely develop worn-down joints.

Heavy Metals Can Cause Inflammation

One marker your doctor can check for in your blood work is the presence of antinuclear antibodies (ANA), which can be associated with mercury-induced autoimmunity. Other heavy metals, like cadmium, have been associated with autoimmune disease, and can also cause ANA-positive blood tests. The ANA-positive test has been associated with many types of autoimmune disease, including lupus and rheumatoid arthritis, and, interestingly, studies support the theory that exposure to low levels of mercury could synergize with other risk factors to promote or exacerbate autoimmune disease.

The American Dental Association reports that 5–10 percent of people are allergic to mercury fillings. We have already discussed how certain heavy metals, like nickel, can cause rashes. An autoimmune reaction to mercury can be quite diverse, especially if it occurs due to dental fillings. The tissue in the mouth is different from the skin, so instead of developing a rash in the mouth it can create a systemic immune response, causing hair loss, joint pain, digestive issues, rashes on other parts of the skin, and even difficulty concentrating. Again, the inflammation will affect your weak spot first.

Fran's Health Was Affected by Toxic Heavy Metals

Fran came to see me for the first time in 2006. She was a fifty-six-year-old woman who was in good health, yet she was concerned about some nagging symptoms that she thought were associated with getting older. She complained of constant fatigue and constipation, and, most importantly, muscle and joint aches in her knees, hands, and feet. She had difficulty sleeping at night, seasonal allergies that caused dry eyes, and she was beginning to experience symptoms of arthritis. She told me that her last menstrual cycle had ended two years ago, and that she supposed her dry eyes were related to menopause.

We decided to run a full workup of blood tests, including for Lyme disease. Because of her specific symptoms, I recommended that we do blood and urine tests for heavy metals like mercury, lead, and cadmium. Her heavy metal tests came back showing a significantly elevated level of lead. The reference range should be under 5, and her levels showed up at 110. In addition, the test for cadmium showed that she had the highest level of the heavy metal I've ever seen.

Because Fran's test results were so high, we decided to treat her with a thorough heavy metal detoxification. We did a comprehensive evaluation of her home environment, including having her water and soil checked for heavy metals. However, we couldn't find any source of exposure. To make things more complicated, her blood tests for cadmium and lead (which would be elevated if there was a current exposure) where always negative. I came to the conclusion that her elevated levels must be from an exposure in her distant past, and that her overall body burden had reached a level where she began to have symptoms.

During the course of heavy metal detoxification, her joint symptoms began to improve and her cadmium and lead levels declined. By 2008 she had significantly fewer joint symptoms, significantly fewer allergy symptoms, and her energy was improving quite a bit. She no longer has dry eyes, joint stiffness, joint pain, or allergy symptoms.

Fran is still seeing me as a patient and her levels of lead and cadmium are still elevated; however, her original symptoms are almost completely gone. She now continues to enjoy her life as much as ever before.

Supplements That Decrease Inflammation

If the symptoms of inflammation do not go away after you have completed your 30-day detox plan, you may want to consider adding certain supplements to help improve how you feel. The supplements can work like natural anti-inflammatory and immune modulators, and thereby raise the threshold for symptoms in your weakest spot. Remember, supplements don't work by themselves; they should be used in conjunction with your meal plan to help you achieve optimal health results. Appendix 1 provides all the information you need about supplements that help combat inflammation.

Improving Detoxification and the Immune Response

It's important to realize that if the immune system is involved in a prolonged or ongoing response, as it continues to fight toxins, the inflammation it creates will slow down the natural detoxification process, which will also adversely affect our health. The following are additional solutions you may want to explore that can further improve the detox process and help bolster your immune system. While by no means mandatory, these modalities can be very beneficial in further improving the workings of the immune system and alleviating related symptoms.

Lymphatic System

DRY BRUSHING

Gently brush your skin with either your hand or a soft-bristled brush, starting at your feet and brushing toward your abdomen; then start again with your fingers and brush toward your neck. You can do this on yourself or you can have it done as part of a specialized massage therapy. This technique improves the circulation of fluid within the lymphatic system, enabling the body to remove toxins storied in lymphatic tissue. This technique is great for reducing swelling in the ankles and hands and is good for improving toxin drainage.

LYMPHATIC DRAINAGE

This technique is performed by a trained therapist who sequentially brushes and massages the skin, starting at your feet and hands and moving toward your abdomen and neck. Devices have been created to improve the effectiveness of this technique, such as the light beam generator, which delivers light over specific lymphatic areas with the goal of improving the function and drainage of the lymphatic system. This technique is great for removing swelling in the arms and legs and for improving toxin drainage.

Lungs

DIAPHRAGM BREATHING

When you strengthen the most important muscle for breathing, the diaphragm, you will be able to maintain superior oxygen levels and efficiently remove carbon dioxide from the body. In this exercise, you move breath up from your belly instead of through your chest. This opens the belly and allows the diaphragm to move deeper down into your abdomen on the inhalation and farther up, to squeeze your lungs and support your heart, on the exhalation.

Lie down on your back on a bed, a yoga mat, or even a carpeted floor. Place your hands one on top of the other on your belly, with the center of your lower hand touching your navel. Focus your breath so that your belly expands as you inhale and retracts as you exhale. If your belly seems tight, lightly massage the outside edge of your belly button. Notice how your belly begins to soften and relax. If your belly does not move as you breathe, press down on it with your hands as you exhale. Then as you inhale, gradually release the tension. Try this several times. Notice how your belly begins to open more on the inhalation. Although it's easiest if you are lying down, you can also practice while you are sitting, standing, or even walking.

ACUPUNCTURE

Acupuncture is a procedure that involves inserting and manipulating needles in various points on the body to relieve pain and for other therapeutic purposes. Traditional Chinese medicine treats the lungs in a way that's quite different from what we are used to in conventional Western medicine. Instead of focusing only on the physical lungs, acupuncture helps to restore proper energy flow to enhance all the supporting organs, so the lungs can detoxify better and be in balance with the rest of the body. Acupuncture is performed in a trained practitioner's office.

Skin

SAUNAS

The sauna is a great way to make use of the excretory organs of the skin to sweat out toxins. The process works by raising your surface body temperature to the ambient temperature of the sauna, which causes you to sweat while maintaining a normal core body temperature of 98.6°F.

A sauna can be installed in your home, or you can access one at a local gym or a day spa. I once treated a patient who completely detoxified herself from mercury by using her home sauna every day for a year.

A Swedish sauna has a temperature range between 160°F and 200°F and is very effective. Do not spend more that twenty minutes in a Swedish sauna at one time or your core body temperature will rise and you will overheat.

Infrared (IR) saunas have a much lower external temperature, between 110°F and 130°F. They work by raising external body temperature and by using a heating element that radiates IR spectrum heat, which is thought to more deeply penetrate your skin and thus provide more thorough detoxification. Because the temperature range is lower in an IR sauna, you can generally stay in longer without overheating.

BATHING IN EPSOM SALT OR SEA SALT

A warm bath in Epsom or sea salt allows you to sweat out toxins with the added benefit of absorbing some of the minerals and trace minerals found in salts. The salts generally contain a considerable amount of magnesium and other trace minerals. If a person is depleted of these minerals, which can happen during saunas, or has difficulty absorbing minerals from food because of poor digestion, or has difficulty retaining minerals because of some underlying health condition, the minerals in these salt baths can be very restorative. The main drawback to using water to detoxify is that water is generally treated or has contaminants like those discussed in chapter 3. Make sure you use filtered water or water that you know has been tested and certified as clear of impurities.

Pour one cup of Epsom salt or sea salt into bathwater that's hot but not too hot for you to sit in comfortably for twenty minutes. Lay down in the bath so that you are covered with water to your lower chest. Place a towel on top of you in the bath. The towel allows you to achieve an even greater level of perspiration in the tub, while also maintaining the water temperature.

EXFOLIATION

Removing the outermost layer of dead skin cells from the face and body is useful for more than just having a youthful appearance; it is also smart to do before detoxifying in a sauna or bath because as you remove the dead layers of skin cells you open the pores in your skin, which will allow sweat and toxins to more easily escape from your body.

You can easily exfoliate your body on a weekly basis in the privacy of your own home. Choose a topical exfoliating scrub or loofah sponge that is specifically designed for your skin type and the part of the body to be exfoliated. You can use a coarser sponge on the body and a very fine scrub for the face.

Brush dry skin before getting into the shower, using a dry loofah sponge, exfoliating gloves, or a body exfoliating brush, starting at the soles of the feet and working your way up, avoiding the genitals and face. Then get into the bath or shower and wet your entire body. Apply exfoliating cleanser to your loofah or exfoliating brush or gloves. Scrub your body using gentle, circular motions.

Look for a natural, organic exfoliating product that contains ingredients such as oatmeal, ground almonds, or even sea salt. The grainy texture exfoliates the skin without harsh chemicals. During the summer it is important to do less exfoliation on the face and exposed areas of your body, so you are not more susceptible to the sun's damaging rays.

MUD AND CLAY PACKS

Packs provide a gentle way to pull impurities and toxins out of the skin. Generally, these treatments can be sought out at spas, but you can also purchase mud and clay masks for home use. To avoid contaminants, look for products that have no additives or fragrances.

BAKING SODA

Baking soda has thousands of uses, including alkalizing bathwater as part of a detoxification bath. Pour one cup of baking soda into bathwater just like you would for a sea salt or Epsom salt bath, and soak for twenty minutes.

Baking soda can also be taken internally and will help detoxify the body by improving your alkalinity. Just mix between one-half and one teaspoon in three ounces of water and drink: this can help with acid reflux and reverse mild allergic reactions, like hives or brain fog, after eating food that you are sensitive to.

As you can see, many symptoms of failing health are related to inflammation and the immune response to toxins. This becomes especially evident as we discuss, in the next few chapters, symptoms that relate to the digestive tract, heart disease, and even hormone balance.

Chapter 9

Resolving Digestion and Weight Issues

Certain types of food are toxic to our digestive system and can not only cause us to gain weight but also strangely influence our future food choices. For example, processed foods and those primarily comprised of simple carbohydrates are both low in nutrients and full of sugar, which can be detrimental to our health and our waistline. It has been clear for some time that excess sugar consumption can lead to binge eating, compulsive eating, food cravings, and sugar addiction. Sugar stimulates the dopamine and opioid receptors of the brain. These are the same receptors that are stimulated by other addictive substances, including drugs like cocaine and morphine, and, just like those drugs, sugar can become habit forming and withdrawal symptoms can develop when consumption is cut back or stopped. Ultimately, the prolonged consumption of an excess of refined sugar in the diet will lead to weight gain and other serious diseases, like type 2 diabetes, heart disease, and stroke. Other chemical toxins affect our weight in a different way. For example, chlorine is an antibiotic that is added to water as a disinfectant, but when we drink chlorinated water, it kills the good bacteria in our digestive tract. That's another reason why filtering chlorinated water is so important.

Having the right balance of good bacteria is critical to proper digestion. Researchers are finding that the types of bacteria found in the digestive tract may be one of the factors determining whether a person will be lean or obese. According to a 2009 article in *Environmental Health Perspectives,* the phylum of bacteria associated with being lean is Bacteroidetes, while the phylum associated with obesity is Firmicutes.

Exactly which bacteria belonging to each of these groups is still being investigated, but what is astonishing is that these bacteria are thought to be affected by environmental factors. For example, if a person is exposed to a high-fat diet or certain environmental toxins or antibiotics, they will be more susceptible to developing gut bacteria of the type associated with obesity. This is the case, for example, with overexposure to chlorinated water. Heavy metals can also affect your internal bacteria. If you are getting exposed to mercury from the fillings in your teeth every time you chew or drink hot liquids, or from eating a diet of large fish like tuna or swordfish, then you may also be causing a shift in your digestive tract toward these bad bacteria.

An excess of bad bacteria can also lead to excess growth of yeast. Not only will excess yeast make digestion uncomfortable (think yeast infection or urinary tract infection), but yeast is a living organism that survives by being fed. The yeast depends on sugar to live and creates toxins that stimulate you to have exaggerated sugar cravings or fall into the trap of binge eating. In the end, excess sugar is your diet downfall. But as you can see, it's your toxic body that makes you reach for that extra cookie and not lack of willpower.

Sugar Is Linked to Inflammation

We know that inflammation caused by an improper immune response can create swelling and fluid retention throughout the body. Inflammation, as we learned in the last chapter, is the body's way of protecting itself from infection and toxins. Usually, the body will have a limited immune response until the offending agent is resolved. For example, you may have a sore throat that lasts about seven to ten days, which goes away when the virus is cleared. However, if your body is producing inflammation in response to something that you are constantly being exposed to, the inflammation will not resolve. Many environmental allergy sufferers know how bad they can feel during the spring, summer, or fall when they are temporarily exposed to pollen from trees, grasses, or weeds. These people often know whether pollen is in the air without the help of the weather report. A person with a cat allergy will know immediately what type of pet is in a home because they will develop itchy eyes as soon as they walk through the door. These are temporary inflammatory responses. However, if you have symptoms of inflammation all the time, then you may be getting exposed to something every day. One of the main reasons for constant exposure is that you are continuously eating a food that you are unknowingly allergic to.

Inflammation can come from food allergies or simply eating the wrong types of food. I believe that every year on a highly processed diet takes about three months off your life. If you are like most Americans, you have cereal with milk for breakfast, maybe a sandwich for lunch, and then some type of protein with pasta or potato and possibly vegetables for dinner. All of these meals are packed with simple sugars. Once you remove the cereal, bread, and pasta from your diet, you may just find that the swelling in your ankles or hands reduces or the excess pounds you always had a problem with finally melt away, because your body is no longer holding on to extra fluid.

The detox diet will help you break the bad habits of relying on simple carbs for fast, filling meals. Instead you will be eating a wide variety of fresh vegetables, fruits, and lean proteins. By doing so, you will be avoiding the toxins, chemicals, and inflammatory foods that have been leaving you feeling tired and bloated. And, as many of my patients report, by the end of the first week you'll have little interest in eating sugar; by the end of the month you may find that you have no interest in returning to your old eating style because you feel so much better with your new food choices.

Preservatives Are Part of the Problem

Processed foods like pizza, fast-food hamburgers, chips, and cereals also contain a great deal of preservatives. Have you ever wondered why you are eating a food that has an expiration date two years from now? Manufacturers of these foods are concerned that bacteria and mold will eat those foods before you will. Food preservatives generally fall into two categories: antimicrobials and antioxidants. The antimicrobials include sulfites and sodium nitrite, and they do exactly what you would expect: they inhibit the growth of mold and bacteria. The antioxidants include BHA and BHT, and they are different from the antioxidants that improve your health. In this instance, they work to prevent cellular oxidation reactions from occurring, which means they prevent cell growth. In your body, these preservatives probably don't cause much harm in small quantities, but if your diet is entirely made up of packaged foods and preserved meats, your body can become toxic from overexposure, and you will experience symptoms of inflammation and fluid retention as your body tries to dilute their concentrations in your blood.

Processed foods are equally dangerous for their lack of ingredients, including essential vitamins, minerals, fiber, and other nutrients that have been stripped out of them. When this happens, these foods lose the proper ratio of good fats to bad fats. If the balance between bad fats (omega-6) and good fats (omega-3) becomes too unbalanced, then you can become more susceptible to inflammation and fluid retention. Ideally, the ratio of omega-6 fats to omega-3 fats should be around two to one, like what is naturally found in wild salmon or grass-fed beef. However, when foods are processed, and the omega-3 fats are destroyed and the omega-6 fats are enhanced by the addition of omega-6 oils like vegetable oils (e.g., soy, safflower, and canola oils), the ratio of omega-6 to omega-3 fats can increase to one hundred to one. Too much omega-6 fatty acid increases inflammation. The good news is that when you follow the detox diet you will automatically restore the beneficial balance of omega-6 to omega-3 fatty acids.

Is Salt Toxic?

Packaged or processed foods also contain high amounts of salt, which can also cause fluid retention. If you are currently trying to control your blood pressure, you may have been put on a low-salt diet. This is because when you develop atherosclerosis, or hardening of the arteries, the blood vessels actually become stiff and inflexible. With excessive salt in the diet, the body will retain water, which puts added pressure on the stiff blood vessels. Because the blood vessels can't flex with the additional water volume, blood pressure elevates. This is almost like trying to add extra air to a fully inflated balloon: each additional breath of air brings the balloon closer to popping. And just like a balloon can burst from being overinflated, our blood vessels can burst from too much fluid, resulting in hemorrhaging (bleeding) and stroke.

When you eat foods that are high in sodium, initially the blood-salt concentration increases and the body compensates by sucking water out of cells in an attempt to restore proper water balance, leaving you feeling bloated and puffy. Your energy will sag because salt causes your cells to become dehydrated, and you may develop muscle cramping, irritability, and mood swings as your dehydrated muscle and brain cells have more difficulty carrying out their routine functions.

However, on the detox diet you will be naturally limiting your salt intake, because you will be eating only fresh fruits, vegetables, and lean protein. By staying away from processed foods, you are giving both your digestive system and your taste buds a break. You'll notice in just a few days that fresh foods have real, delicious, distinct tastes, instead of just salty or sweet.

Sylvia Detoxed, Lost 17 Pounds, and Kept Them Off

Sylvia was seventy-seven when she first came to see me in 2008. Her chief complaints were fatigue and memory changes. Sylvia believed that she was in good health, except that she thought she might have low thyroid function because her energy was dwindling. She also had begun to notice that she was becoming forgetful, but she attributed her brain fog to the stress she was under: her husband had been recently diagnosed with Alzheimer's disease and his health was failing.

While Sylvia had no medical history, and was not taking any prescription medications, her total score on the detox questionnaire was 90 (remember, the goal is 14 or lower). I told Sylvia that although she didn't have many symptoms, something was wrong with her health. Her high score may have been caused by her diet. I explained to her that certain processed foods can become very habit forming because of the amount of sugar in them, and Sylvia realized that her diet did in fact contain lots of processed foods.

We decided to also do a hormone workup for her, checking thyroid and sex hormones, and we discussed starting the detox diet while we waited to get the results of the blood work. Sylvia was enthusiastic about the diet program because she had a history of food addiction and had struggled with her weight for her entire life. She thought that the detox, based on two shakes a day plus snacks and a healthy dinner, would give her the structure she was looking for.

I saw Sylvia again about six weeks later, and she was happy to report that she was feeling better. She felt significantly more clearheaded and was having more-regular bowel movements, less-achy muscles and joints, and she was feeling more emotionally stable. Her questionnaire score went from 90 to 32. Even more impressive, her weight changed from 184 pounds to 179. Sylvia was particularly proud of this because she had told me that she had not been able to lose weight with any other meal plan in the past.

The blood work came back very positive, aside from a hormone imbalance. We talked about bioidentical hormone-replacement therapy, and I started her on a very low dose of topical estrogen and progesterone. When I asked her to schedule a follow-up appointment in two months, Sylvia asked if she could remain on the detox diet. I told her that if she was getting good results, she could stay on without reintroducing foods until our next appointment.

By the end of 2008, Sylvia told me that she was "feeling wonderful." She's was more centered and felt the detox meal plan helped her a great deal with appetite control and food addiction, and that the hormone replacement therapy was giving her better energy. She started to exercise and decided to stay on the detox diet until she reached her goal weight. Now, two years later, her weight has stabilized at 167 pounds and her total detox questionnaire score is 5.

Xenoestrogens Affect Weight Gain

It has now been scientifically proven that chemicals impact hormone receptors in the body, which can force metabolism to slow down, causing weight gain as the body learns to hoard calories rather than burn them. Xenoestrogens, or hormone-mimicking pollutants, ubiquitous in the food chain, have been shown to act on genes during early childhood, enhancing the development of fat cells, which stay with you for life. Retha Newbold of the National Institute of Environmental Health Sciences in North Carolina, part of the National Institutes of Health, believes, as I do, that there is plenty of evidence showing that being overweight is not just the result of personal choices about what you eat combined with inactivity. Exposure to environmental chemicals during development may be contributing to the obesity epidemic.

That's right, environmental chemicals may well account for a good part of the current epidemic, especially for those under fifty years old. Paula Baillie-Hamilton, MD, at Stirling University in Scotland, first reported in the *Journal of Alternative and Complementary Medicine* in 2002 that obesity rates had risen with the use of chemicals such as pesticides and plasticizers over the past forty years. Scientists in Japan also found that low levels of certain compounds, such as bisphenol A (used in baby bottles), had surprising effects on cells growing in lab dishes. They found that cells that would typically become fibroblasts, or connective-tissue cells, were instead changing into adipocytes, or fat cells. The same toxins also stimulated the proliferation of existing fat cells. In 2005 scientists in Spain reported that the more pesticides children were exposed to as fetuses, the greater their risk of being overweight as toddlers.

In 2006 another study, conducted by Bruce Blumberg of the University of California, Irvine, showed that pregnant mice fed tributyltin, a disinfectant and fungicide used in marine paints, plastics production, and other products, which enters the food chain in seafood and drinking water, produced offspring that were born with more stored fat, more fat cells, and became 5–20 percent fatter by adulthood. The tributyltin activated a switch that determined the cells' fate: in one position it allowed cells to remain fibroblasts, in another it guided them to become fat cells. Blumberg named these compounds, including some phthalates, bisphenol A, and perfluoroalkyl compounds (used in stain repellents and nonstick cooking surfaces) "obesogens" because their reaction was so consistent.

In January 2009 scientists in Belgium found that children exposed to higher levels of PCBs and DDT before birth were fatter than those exposed to lower levels. Clearly it is not a coincidence that the obesity rate in our country is connected to the amount of xenoestrogens and estrogen-like chemicals that we are exposed to. Following the detox diet and making the lifestyle changes needed to diminish or eliminate exposure to these chemicals will give you a chance to regain the optimal health you know you can achieve.

Toxins Also Cause Weight Loss

All of this data is particularly interesting because in the past toxic exposure was thought to cause weight loss instead of weight gain. This was especially true for people who had continuous, high-level exposures, which would impact them by causing decreased appetite, nausea, or other digestive dysfunctions like chronic diarrhea and would potentially lead to death if the exposure was not discovered in time. However, these conditions only happened to people who worked in the chemical industry and had regular, albeit accidental, high-level exposures.

My primary concern is for those of us who are getting low-level chronic or intermittent exposures that are not enough to cause appetite suppression and other lethal health effects but instead lead to weight gain and other nonlethal symptoms, which might include fatigue and a general sense of poor health.

CLEANING AND COOKING FISH TO REMOVE TOXINS

PCBs, dioxins, mirex, DDT, chlordane, and dieldrin are found at high levels in the fat of fish. You can reduce the amount of these contaminants by properly trimming, skinning, and cooking fresh fish. First remove and discard all the skin and trim all the fat from the belly flap and the rest of the fish body. Cut away a V-shaped wedge to remove the dark fatty tissue along the entire length of the fillet.

Toxins and Digestive Tract Issues

Chlorine and fluoride are lethal to cells in high concentrations. Even at low levels, however, these chemicals act as disinfectants and pesticides. When they are added to water in small concentrations for disinfecting purposes, they can, over time, destroy the balance of good bacteria in the digestive tract, causing symptoms that include bloating, constipation, and loose bowel movements. A more common cause of digestive symptoms can be toxic parasites.

The following symptoms can be tracked to specific exposures:

Bloating, belching, passing gas: Excess gas production in the digestive tract can be related to the fermentation of food from excess yeast or methane-producing bad bacteria.

Constipation: Occurs because of a lack of good bacteria in the digestive tract. These bacteria form up to 60 percent of the dry mass of bowel movements. Constipation also develops due to dehydration from excessive salt consumption or from inadequate fiber in the diet.

Diarrhea: Occurs from excess bad bacteria or parasites in the digestive tract, which cause inflammation and the inability to properly absorb fluids from stool. It can also develop from rapid transit of stool as the body tries to eliminate harmful bad bacteria. If loose stools persist or there is blood or mucus in the stool, see your doctor immediately so he can determine if you have a parasite or other health condition that may require special attention.

Heartburn, indigestion, or reflux: These typically occur if there is inflammation in the stomach due to infection, such as from *H. pylori*. It can also be a sign of inadequate digestive enzymes, which are necessary to trigger reflexive shutting of the lower esophageal sphincter (the connection between the esophagus and the stomach).

Intestinal/stomach pain, nausea, vomiting: All are symptoms of irritation and inflammation of the digestive tract, which can develop from infections or food allergies that cause intestinal cramping.

Don't Create a New Home for Parasites

There are ten times more foreign bacteria in our digestive tract than there are cells in our entire body. These good bacteria, when in balance, aid with many body functions, including digestion, absorption, and immunity. However, if the good bacteria become unbalanced, which can happen if you pick up a parasite, you will have health problems.

Despite the fact that we live in a first-world country, and generally believe that we do not get exposed to parasites, the fact is that parasites don't know borders and exist within the United States. Many types of parasitic organisms live off us and adversely affect our health. Microscopic parasites can cause an immune response that leads to inflammation in the digestive tract and throughout the body. This particular type of inflammation can cause digestive symptoms, including any of those listed above as well as food cravings. If you have an insatiable appetite despite eating well-balanced meals, or if you feel that you are constantly craving sugar, bread, or dairy products, or have chronic rectal itching, you may have a parasite.

Parasites can create inflammation in the digestive tract, causing diarrhea and abdominal cramping when you are first exposed to the infection. However, if you don't treat the parasite when you first get it, or if it is not treated completely, you can develop a chronic, persistent carrier state in which you have a low-level infection causing persistent digestive problems that don't resolve with diet modification.

Many parasites enter our body from eating raw food, particularly from sushi and salad bars. Nonsymptomatic migrant workers can be carriers of parasites and introduce them from all over the world into our local food chain. The parasites not only cause digestive issues but produce their own toxins that can affect your health and add to your body burden. So the problem with parasites is not only the infection, inflammation, and immune response but also the chemicals they produce that become an extra toxic burden for our body.

If you have a mildly weak digestive tract because you have been taking antacids, antibiotics, or steroids, you can be susceptible to infections from parasites. This is because these medicines can decrease the acidity in the stomach and handicap our first and most important line of defense from these organisms.

Chronic digestive issues can mean that you have bad bacteria or too much yeast in your digestive tract. We know that inflammation and digestive symptoms can come from having an infection in the digestive tract. Sometimes chronic carriers of parasites are incorrectly diagnosed with irritable bowel syndrome and end up experiencing either constipation or loose bowel movements, or cramping and indigestion symptoms, all of which would resolve if the parasite was discovered and treated appropriately.

In this day and age, it's a lot easier for parasites to get into our body. Besides living in a global marketplace, our bodies have changed so that parasites are more welcome and stay longer. For example, as mentioned, the acid produced in the stomach is the first line of defense against invading parasites. The pH of the stomach is literally supposed to be 2, which is super acidic—akin to hydrochloric acid and able to kill most foreign bacteria and parasites. Yet if you are under a lot of stress, your stomach acid pH will become weaker. When people get reflux or other digestive symptoms, doctors readily prescribe antacids to take away those symptoms. But as a consequence, the pH in the stomach becomes even more alkaline, so the antacids actually end up taking away our first line of defense. This is one of the reasons why some people who were once able to tolerate raw foods are now susceptible to the microscopic organisms that may be found on them. The invaders are getting past that first line of defense and into the digestive tract to set up shop.

You can get rid of parasites when you modify your diet. By removing dairy products, wheat, and sugar, all of which decrease stomach acidity and weaken the immune system, you will lower the likelihood of parasites entering your digestive tract. I would council against eating too many raw foods, especially if you are taking prescription medications that affect your digestive function. Pay close attention to the "possible side effects" of many prescription and over-the-counter medications to see if they are affecting your digestion.

When you follow the detox diet, you will be automatically taking stress off your body, which will improve your digestive function. You will be avoiding the foods that weaken your immune system, cause inflammation, and decrease stomach acidity, and you will be avoiding the chemicals that destroy good bacteria in the digestive tract. At the same time you will be strengthening your digestive function by choosing foods that actually improve digestion.

Supplementing your diet with good bacteria like acidophilus and bifidobacillus can help push bad bacteria out of the digestive tract. Eating bitter foods like wasabi, horseradish, radishes, arugula, and kale can help improve stomach acid pH and hydrochloric acid production. In severe cases, prescription medications may be necessary to eradicate parasites. If you believe this may be a problem you are dealing with, it's important to work with your health care provider to get the correct prescription medications if necessary.

Mary Fae's Stomach Pains Resolved on the Detox Diet

Mary Fae came to my office when she was twenty-eight. Even though she felt that she was in good health, her digestive gas, bloating, and reflux would not go away. She had tried every remedy on the market for more than ten years, with little relief. At first she went the conventional route with medications and antacids, but it never helped. She had no major medical problems other than the reflux, and when she saw me, she was off her prescription medications. Her previous doctor had recommended an endoscopy six months before, which just showed gastritis, or inflammation of the stomach. During our first meeting, she weighed in at 159, and her initial detox questionnaire showed an overall score of 98 (the goal is 14 or below). Otherwise, her physical exam was normal.

Mary Fae told me that she had been able to manage her symptoms with portion control, but over the past year her symptoms had become worse, with more gas and bloating, pain, and reflux, regardless of when she had eaten. So we checked for food allergies and parasites. We also did a blood test for *H. pylori*. Because her questionnaire score was relatively high, I started her immediately on the detox diet. I also started her on probiotics and digestive enzymes I thought might help her stomach improve digestion, rather than impede digestion, as occurs with prescription acid blockers.

Her second visit, three weeks later, found Mary Fae in a much better mood. She came into my office with a smile and told me that since she'd been on the detox diet she'd had a lighter menstrual cycle, less acne, and, most important, less gas and bloating. Her score on the detox questionnaire dropped from 98 to 39, and her weight went from 159 pounds to 149.

It turned out that she had an excessive amount of yeast in her digestive tract. Her food-allergy test showed that she had a clear sensitivity to dairy products. Mary Fae said that she was feeling so much better by eliminating dairy from her diet that she wanted to stay on the detox diet until the next visit.

Six weeks later, Mary Fae came in with more energy, even less pain with her menstrual cycle, and less bloating. And she also discovered that when she ate cucumbers or anything with apple cider vinegar, she would get abdominal pain. Her questionnaire score now dropped to 20 and her weight was down another 10 pounds, to 139.

At that point, we made a decision to try reintroducing foods to her diet because she was feeling so much better. Interestingly, she had discovered on her own, while following the detox diet, that cucumbers and apple cider vinegar caused her symptoms of reflux and abdominal gas and bloating. This was particularly interesting because typically, I tell my patients to use apple cider vinegar to help improve stomach symptoms, but in Mary Fae's case, it made things worse. We speculated that the symptoms came on either because she was allergic to those foods or because there was some chemical in those foods that her body was not able to tolerate properly. She learned that as long as she avoids those foods and dairy, she feels quite a bit better.

When we modified Mary Fae's diet to decrease the stimulus to yeast by removing sugar and dairy products, and put her on probiotics like acidophilus that helped replace the yeast with good bacteria, her body was able to help itself. When the underlying problems were removed, her symptoms improved.

The Importance of Fiber

Fiber is a very important part of our diet, especially during the 30-day detox. Fiber, or roughage, is the undigestible, unabsorbed part of vegetables that helps give the stool form and consistency. Nutritional science has extolled the benefits of fiber for years, and at this point it is clear that consuming twenty to thirty grams of fiber daily can decrease the risk of heart disease, diabetes, and colon cancer, while at the same time improving bowel regularity and the detox process.

Fiber can be split into two categories: soluble and insoluble. Soluble fiber attracts and holds on to water, bile salts, and cholesterol. It also binds toxins, which makes it an essential part of the 30-day detox diet, allowing the toxins your body is trying to expel to be transported out of your body with your bowel movement. You can find soluble fiber in oat bran (which you should avoid if you are on a gluten-free diet), flaxseed, psyllium husk, and fruit pectin.

Insoluble fiber passes through our intestines largely intact and helps to maintain a healthy stool transit time of about twelve to eighteen hours after eating. Insoluble fiber can be found in vegetables, fruit, root vegetable skin, nuts, and seeds. During your detox diet, you should get your insoluble fiber only from vegetables, fruits, and root vegetable skins, while avoiding nuts and seeds during the first month at least, especially if weight loss is a goal.

It is very important to have at least one to three bowel movements daily. This allows your body to remove toxins before they have an opportunity to get reabsorbed in your digestive tract. If you find that you are not achieving this level of regularity, you may want to try following some of the supplement recommendations listed in appendix 1 under improving digestive regularity.

BITTER HERBS

Bitter herbs are a natural way to treat digestive issues. For example, radishes can help treat heartburn. Fresh garlic can be a remedy for the common cold. Garlic is really great as a natural antibiotic—it kills infections.

Improving Weight Loss and Digestion

The following are some solutions you may want to explore to further improve your digestion and enhance weight loss. While not mandatory, these modalities can be very beneficial to your digestive system and effective in alleviating related symptoms.

Liver and the Digestive Tract

Colonic Hydrotherapy

This technique is very useful for more than just chronic constipation, it is also important for improving detoxification by stimulating the reflexive dumping of toxins as stool is eliminated from the body. Low-pressure water is administered into the large intestine by a trained colonic therapist with the goal of both removing impacted or retained stool from the entire colon as well as enhancing the transit time in which bile produced by the gallbladder is evacuated.

Bile is full of enzymes that help to digest fat, and it contains many toxins as well. Under ordinary circumstances, the bile will move through the colon with digested food in a process that generally takes twelve to twenty-four hours. During that time, most of the bile is reabsorbed for reprocessing in the body. However, a good portion of the toxins get reabsorbed as well. During a successful colonic therapy session, the transit time is increased to about forty-five to sixty minutes, thereby allowing the body to evacuate whatever toxins were in the bile.

When this is done properly, my patients report a feeling of clear headedness and a light feeling in the body. Colonics should not be performed more than once a week because they can cause depletion of fluids and vitamins, which can lead to sleepiness and irritability. There are a great number of colon-cleansing products on the market, made to be used at home, with the implied purpose of improving detoxification through improved colon function. While these products may be beneficial, I suggest that you check with your health care provider before using them, because they should be used along with a program that includes diet and lifestyle modification.

Vitamin C Flush (a.k.a. Vitamin C Calibration)

Vitamin C is a water-soluble vitamin that, when taken orally, has a maximum range of absorption: after absorbing a certain amount the body eliminates the excess. Most people can take about six thousand milligrams before the absorption capacity is reached. After the maximum dose is achieved, the vitamin C will pull body fluids into the colon and you will experience a loose, watery bowel movement, which is beneficial to detoxification because, just like with colonic therapy, toxins are more rapidly transported out of the body through the digestive tract.

Finding out how much vitamin C you need gives you an idea of your antioxidant requirements. Some people find they need less vitamin C to create a flush, which suggests that their body has adequate antioxidant protection. Others find they require more vitamin C, which suggests that their body requires a significant amount of antioxidants for their health condition. The more vitamin C you require, the more likely it is that you have a health problem adversely affecting your body.

A vitamin C flush takes approximately one day. It is best to start on an empty stomach, first thing in the morning. Dissolve a half teaspoon (1.5 grams) of L-ascorbate powder in two or more ounces of water. After dissolving and allowing any effervescence to abate (typically within two minutes), drink the beverage. Count and record each dosage. Follow with a level half teaspoon dissolved in one to two ounces of water every fifteen minutes until you achieve a watery bowel movement. Do not stop when there are just loose stools. You want to energize the body to flush out toxins and reduce the risk that they may recirculate and induce problems. Once the stools are watery, stop consuming the buffered ascorbate for the day. For more information, visit the Web site Perque.com (www.perque.com).

Kidneys

Drainage Remedies

Your health care provider may prescribe products that improve kidney drainage. These are natural remedies created from potent herbal extracts made from plant shoots, leaves, and flowers. This technique was first developed in the early 1900s as a way of improving the body's ability to heal itself. Some of the remedies are extracts of herbs or just very dilute essences of the original herb. I recommend drainage remedies from the brands Soluna, Pekana, and Heel because they are very gentle and effective for improving kidney detoxification.

When taking these types of remedies, you might notice that you need to urinate more frequently, which is a good sign that your body is healing itself and beginning to pass toxins out more efficiently.

Your chronic digestive symptoms may be affecting your ability to lose weight on diet programs. I strongly believe that the 30-day detox will help you get your digestive system moving so you can finally experience lasting weight loss as well as the alleviation of your digestive symptoms. By eliminating toxins and radically changing your diet, you will be able to not only feel better, but look better.

Chapter 10
Reversing Cardiovascular Disease and Diabetes

When we are young, our cells are rapidly dividing and developing, so we can tolerate a lot of exposure before developing symptoms from toxins in the environment. Back in college, you may have been able to go out for three nights of partying in a row, go to classes every morning, and still function at a reasonably good level. But by the time you enter the workforce, one night out could ruin you for the whole week. This doesn't happen just because you are getting older, but also because you are becoming exposed to toxins and heavy metals in the environment. Or you may be eating a diet of processed foods high in sugar and refined carbohydrates that is poor in the vitamins, minerals, and antioxidants needed for your body to be thorough in its own detoxification processes. In either case, your body's inability to detoxify can create symptoms that typically affect people older than you—you are literally old before your time. Nowhere is this more evident than in cardiovascular symptoms or those related to diabetes.

Diabetes and cardiovascular disease are actually two closely related conditions that both have devastating impacts on health and longevity. Each is caused by distinct types of toxins, and often one of these diseases leads to the other. When combined with obesity, they form a triad of lethal diseases called metabolic syndrome. Luckily, the best way to treat all of these disorders starts with reversing bad habits and a thorough detox.

Inflammation and Heart Disease

Earlier in this book you learned about how toxins accumulate in your body tissue. And as much as your body tries to get rid of them through the normal routes of detoxification, it can reach a point where it just can't handle any more. When this happens, these toxins become stuck inside tissue and inflammation occurs. If you are experiencing the symptoms in group 4 of the questionnaire, your inflammation may be occurring in the cardiovascular system.

Your heart responds to an electrical impulse that triggers every heartbeat. When you are healthy, your heart makes about sixty to ninety beats per minute at rest, circulating up to five liters of blood throughout your body every minute. The blood moves through your blood vessels without much resistance because the blood vessels are wide-open, pliable tubes, almost like the inner tube of a tire. Oxygenated blood travels from the lungs to the rest of the body through your arteries. Remember, oxygen is necessary to drive the efficient, aerobic production of ATP. This means that oxygen is necessary to create energy. After your blood circulates to your tissues, the oxygen is unloaded into your cells' mitochondria, and the deoxygenated blood returns to the heart through veins to begin the process again.

When the heart is not functioning properly, you can start to develop the following symptoms:

- chest pain
- frequent illness
- irregular or skipped heartbeat
- rapid or pounding heartbeat

- shortness of breath
- weakness

If you are experiencing any of these symptoms, it is very important for you to work with your doctor to find the cause. Heart disease is the number one health problem for both women and men in the United States. Almost seven hundred thousand people die of heart disease in the United States each year, yet it is relatively preventable. The occurrence of heart disease can be greatly reduced by taking steps to control the adverse factors that put people at greater risk, which is what this chapter will cover. Risk factors include diet and toxins, and, in particular, improper elimination of toxic metals from the body.

There are many different types of heart conditions, and each may have a toxic component. These include the following:

- **Heart arrhythmia:** A defect in the electrical activity of the heart that can be caused by poor oxygen flow and may be linked to exposure to toxic metals.
- **Coronary artery disease:** This is when the oxygen-carrying arteries develop poor blood flow to the heart. This can develop slowly over time from the development of cholesterol plaque or due to inflammation in the blood vessels caused by excessive sugar or toxins in your diet. If not diagnosed and treated correctly, this can lead to a heart attack.
- **Hypertension (high blood pressure):** This occurs when the arteries become stiff and nonpliable. Instead of performing like the inner tube of a tire, they perform more like a straw. At rest this may not be a problem, but when exercising or under stress, the heart rate rises and the blood vessels carry a significant larger volume of blood. The larger volume can exceed the capacity of the blood vessels to carry the blood. This condition can lead to a rupture of a blood vessel, which can cause a stroke or heart attack. Hypertension has been associated with excessive lead stored in the body.

Toxic Sugar and Diabetes

Sugar is toxic not just to our cells, as we discussed in chapter 5, but to our entire body. The best way to understand the impact excess sugar consumption can have is to take a close look at type 2 diabetes, a condition that occurs when the body cannot create enough insulin and the sugar levels in the blood become elevated.

After eating each and every meal, your body digests the foods and breaks them down into their building blocks: protein, fat, and the sugar molecule glucose. Then your intestines absorb these nutrients and transfer them into the bloodstream, either to be used immediately in producing energy or driving cellular processes, or to be stored. Protein is stored in muscle, fat is stored in body fat, and sugar is stored in the liver. However, if your diet contains too much sugar, the liver's storage capacity can be exceeded and the excess sugar gets stored as fat. The kicker here is that fat and sugar can't be stored unless there is insulin. Insulin is a type of growth hormone that allows for the storage of glucose in the liver as glycogen and the storage of fat in fat cells, and it prevents fat from breaking down. Insulin is only produced when there is sugar in the bloodstream. Under ideal conditions, insulin will escort the sugar out of the blood into insulin-sensitive tissues and into the muscle to use for energy, or to the liver for short-term storage, or into fat cells for long-term storage for later use.

Our blood sugar will rise with different intensity depending on the type of carbohydrates eaten and the type of meal that accompanies the carbohydrates. Complex carbohydrates like whole grains, beans, and squash break down into sugar slowly. This is also true when a carbohydrate is consumed with a protein and fat. Alternatively, simple carbohydrates and processed foods, like white bread, chips, white rice, processed cereal, and fruit and vegetable juices, turn into glucose quickly and are absorbed by the digestive tract and then into the bloodstream rapidly. This quick absorption causes a rapid elevation in blood-sugar levels, which is balanced by the release of larger amounts of insulin from the pancreas to meet the body's need.

If you have difficulty losing weight, you may be producing too much insulin every time you have a processed carbohydrate or sugary meal. If you maintain a high carbohydrate diet, your body is constantly battling to balance blood sugar and insulin, and then storing the excess sugar in body fat. With a high carbohydrate diet, your insulin levels continue to stimulate your liver to store sugar as glycogen, which can cause the liver to enlarge with the tremendous accumulation of glycogen. This process can lead to a condition called fatty liver, which is just what it sounds like: your liver becomes fatty, which inhibits its ability to properly process toxins.

Eventually, the balance between sugar and insulin becomes dysfunctional, and your body may become insulin resistant: the insulin-sensitive cells in the muscle and fat become nonresponsive. They have been completely engorged with more sugar than they can handle, and they are literally trying to protect themselves from the toxicity of sugar. As a consequence, the pancreas needs to release increasing amounts of insulin into the bloodstream to get the same blood-sugar-balancing effect. When this happens, the amount of insulin released with each sugary meal increases, and the detrimental effects from increasing insulin release begin to take effect.

Insulin resistance does not happen overnight. This process can slowly develop over decades as the body tries to protect itself from the adverse affects of excessively high sugar. I believe that the body recognizes sugar as a toxin and tries to keep it from poisoning its inner working by forcing insulin to reach ever-higher amounts before allowing sugar to be chaperoned into the cells.

Because of the widespread overuse of sugar in our society, some people are literally eating their way toward diabetes. If you have a family history of insulin sensitivity, you have a greater risk of developing type 2 diabetes from eating a diet that's high in processed foods and simple carbohydrates. In addition, the toxic effects of excess sugar and the growth-promoting effects of insulin stimulate more than an enlarged liver and fat gain around your midsection. The elevated levels of sugar cause the kidneys to become toxic and lose function, a condition called nephropathy. The elevated blood-sugar levels also impact the immune system, causing increased susceptibility to infections and poor wound healing. The nerve endings in the hands and feet can become toxic and lose perception of touch and pain, a condition called neuropathy. The blood vessels in the eyes can grow inappropriately, stimulated by excessive insulin production, a condition called retinopathy. And the blood vessels in the heart can become inflamed and dysfunctional, leading to heart disease.

Metabolic Syndrome Links Heart Disease to Diabetes

Diabetes and heart disease are closely related medical conditions: patients with diabetes are significantly more likely to develop heart disease than people who do not have diabetes. Additionally, over 70 percent of deaths among patients with diabetes are directly attributable to heart disease.

This conjunction of heart disease and diabetes is now referred to as metabolic syndrome, which entails a constellation of different symptoms that point to the risk of developing diabetes and heart disease because of the effects of insulin and sugar on your metabolism. These symptoms are now becoming recognized as a side effect of the inflammatory process precipitated from the toxic effect of consuming processed, high-sugar foods. These symptoms include the following:

- Elevated triglycerides: >150 mg/dl
- Low HDL cholesterol: < 40 mg/dl (males), < 50 mg/dl (females)
- Elevated blood pressure: >130/85 mmHg
- Elevated fasting blood sugar: >100 mg/dl
- Elevated BMI (body mass index): >30 kg/m^2

Cardiovascular Inflammation and Environmental Toxins

While cholesterol still remains an important risk factor for developing heart disease, inflammation occurring inside of blood vessels is now thought to be an even more important risk factor. This inflammation can be related to the inflammatory effects of excessive sugar in the diet or from environmental toxins—in particular, toxic metals.

The types of toxic metals that can be considered as possible sources of cardiovascular inflammation include mercury, lead, and iron. These heavy metals cause inflammation and injury to the cardiovascular system both because they cause oxidation in our cells, as we discussed in chapter 6, and because their shape allows them to interfere with biological processes driven by similarly shaped nutritional minerals, like calcium, magnesium, zinc, or selenium.

For example, calcium is very important in activating muscle contractions, and magnesium is a mineral that is essential to inactivate, or relax, a muscle contraction. If these minerals are out of balance, then you might experience a muscle cramp. While there are other reasons for muscles to cramp, including dehydration or a depletion of electrolytes like sodium and potassium, if you have ever experienced chronic muscle cramps that don't resolve with increasing your fluids, you may have an imbalance of calcium and magnesium. Calcium is stored in our bones, but magnesium has no long-term storage compartment in the body: it must be constantly replenished through diet. However, as we discussed in chapter 3, nonorganic farming practices have virtually depleted magnesium from the soil and the foods we eat. Both of these important nutrients can be taken as a supplement. See appendix 1 for recommended doses.

The heart is also a muscle, and if your calcium and magnesium levels are out of balance, you will also have problems with heart function. Heavy metals affect the balance of these minerals by interfering with the minerals' ability to bind with heart-muscle mineral-binding sites and can contribute to improper function.

In addition, heavy metals create free radicals and inflammation, and cause cells to age prematurely. By lowering the levels of heavy metals or by increasing the amount of certain good minerals, we can lower inflammation and decrease our risk of heart disease.

Elevated levels of iron can also create inflammation in the body. Keep in mind that iron is a mineral, not a heavy metal. If it is found in the body in the correct range, it can help prevent anemia, but if it is excessively elevated, the risk for heart disease increases. A 2010 study in the *Journal of Vascular Surgery* showed that ferritin levels (a mark of iron storage in the body) correlated with hs-CRP (the blood marker for inflammation in blood vessels) and heart disease. Iron is naturally found in red meat and green leafy vegetables. The body tries to maintain the correct amount of iron by removing the excess through the liver. Some people have a hereditary susceptibility to retaining iron, a condition called hemochromatosis. Men are typically more likely to develop elevated iron stores in the body. Women lose excessive iron every month during their menstrual cycle. However, anyone who cannot remove excess iron has an increased risk of developing heart disease as well as liver toxicity and liver damage. A good way to reduce your iron load is to donate blood through your local hospital or Red Cross.

Zinc is another important mineral for preventing heart disease. Zinc is an essential mineral for proper immune system function, and it helps create sex hormones. It is also necessary for removing heavy metals from their binding sites. A 2010 article in the *American Journal of Clinical Nutrition* showed that a supplement of 45 milligrams of zinc daily is thought to be protective against heart disease and to help prevent inflammation.

Any Lead in Your Body May Be Unsafe

When lead was removed from gasoline and house paint several decades ago, the average person's blood-lead level dropped dramatically. But our levels of lead are still a great deal higher than those of people who lived before the industrial age. That's because we continue to be exposed to lead in our soil and water, as well as from our own bones, where it is stored once it's introduced into our system. Today, nearly 40 percent of all Americans may have blood-lead levels high enough to cause heart problems. A 2003 article in the *Journal of the American Medical Association* examined two thousand women between the ages of forty and fifty-nine, and found that high blood pressure in postmenopausal women is strongly correlated to blood-lead levels. This is because bones break down faster during menopause, releasing stored lead and injuring blood vessels, which leads to high blood pressure.

Fifty years ago, the average blood-lead levels were about 40 mg/dl. The level considered "safe" by the government has continued to fall and is now considered to be less than 10 mg/dl. But a 2006 study published in the medical journal *Circulation*, involving almost fourteen thousand participants over twelve years (from the National Health and Nutrition Examination Survey), questions the idea that any level of this toxic metal is safe. Researchers found that a blood-lead level of over 2 mg/dl caused dramatic increases in heart attacks, strokes, and death. Even after controlling for all other risk factors, including cholesterol, high blood pressure, smoking, and inflammation, the researchers found that the risk of death in people with a blood-lead level that high increased by 25 percent. Deaths from heart disease increased by 55 percent, risk of heart attacks increased by 151 percent, and risk of stroke increased by 89 percent.

Elevated blood-lead levels can suggest either a current low-level exposure from an external source or the release of lead stored in the body from bone turnover. Ultimately, if you have elevated blood lead you need to find out where it is coming from and eliminate the source of exposure.

EASY STEPS TO REDUCE YOUR LEAD EXPOSURE

- Have a "no shoes in the house" policy. A great deal of lead can be tracked into your house in the dust on the soles of shoes. If you suspect that you have lead in your soil, or you work in a business that may expose you to lead (such as if you do welding or you are a plumber), leaving your shoes at the door helps reduce the amount of contamination in your home.
- Take 1,000 mg of buffered vitamin C a day. This helps remove lead from the body.
- Take 2,000 to 4,000 IU of vitamin D_3 a day to prevent your bones from releasing lead into your bloodstream.

A Heart-Healthy Diet Needs to Be Mercury Free

If you are making diet modifications to improve heart health, then your attempts to eat healthfully may actually be making you sicker. We've been told to reduce meat consumption for better heart health and to eat lots of fish due to their beneficial omega-3 fatty acids. Yet when we increase our fish consumption, we may be inadvertently increasing our exposure to mercury. As we discussed in chapter 3, large ocean fish and even farm-raised fish can increase our exposure to mercury. Better options are to eat 100% grass-fed beef, which has as much omega-3 fatty acid as wild salmon. Or choose smaller fish (ones that can fit on your plate whole) like, sardines, herring, or red snapper.

Jerry Reversed High Blood Pressure When He Detoxed

Jerry first came to my office when he was forty-three years old. He knew that he already had high blood pressure, but he wasn't taking any medication. Jerry also told me that his work was very stressful. He worked on Wall Street, and he said that he felt that his job was "aging him." His primary care doctor was concerned about his blood pressure, especially because he was so young, and he felt that Jerry should start taking a beta-blocker. Jerry came to see me because he was looking for another, less-drastic option for controlling his blood pressure.

When he first came in, Jerry's blood pressure was 140/90 (the goal is under 120/70). His weight was 255 pounds. He was six foot one, and his total detox questionnaire score was 27 (the goal is 14 or under). He also was having digestive symptoms including gas and bloating. His energy and his libido were low. He had muscle and joint achiness. After a thorough checkup and blood work that included tests for his cardiac risk factors, I suggested that he start the detox diet to see if it would help with his symptoms.

After one month of following the plan, Jerry returned to my office. He was happy to report that his energy was better. His questionnaire score dropped from 27 to 11 and his weight went from 255 pounds to 234. His blood pressure went from 140/90 to 130/80.

We reviewed his lab results, which showed that he had a very high, random insulin level, which means that he was insulin resistant and very likely on the way to becoming diabetic. His ferritin level, which is a marker of inflammation in the blood vessels, was 550 (an optimal level is under 150). His cholesterol was 234 and his triglycerides were 522. Cholesterol should be under 200 and triglycerides under 100. His HDL was 31, when it should be above 50. His LDL could not be calculated because his triglycerides were so high. Jerry clearly had the signs of metabolic syndrome, and if he didn't do something about his diet and lifestyle, he was going to have hypertension, heart disease, and diabetes. He felt that if he continued on the detox diet, he would continue to see good results.

I saw Jerry again a month later, and he said that his energy continued to be very good. His blood pressure dropped to 120/70, which is considered normal. After three months of following the diet, we rechecked his blood. We found his fasting blood sugar to be in the normal range. His cholesterol dropped to 171 without prescription medications. His triglyceride levels went from 522 to 78. His HDL levels went from 31 to

54, and now his LDL level could be calculated and it was 102, which is basically normal. His fasting insulin level also became normal.

Jerry still comes to see me. At his most recent visit, a little bit over a year after his first, he felt like he was doing great. He had no complaints. He was still not taking any prescription medications. His weight stabilized at 209 pounds, down significantly from 255 when he started, and his blood pressure has remained in an acceptably normal range.

Jerry is a perfect example of how you should not settle for believing that getting older means living with symptoms. Fatigue, high blood pressure, and weight gain are not symptoms of aging but of lifestyle. Remember, the body is constantly trying to heal itself, and if we give it the right environment, it will do just that. Our job is to give our body the opportunity, the right building blocks, and the right foundation. In this case, Jerry needed to lower his body burden by getting rid of toxins and to give his body all the nutrients it needed to heal itself. Like Jerry, you have control over your healing process.

Improving Cardiovascular and Metabolic Function

The following are other solutions you may want to explore to further improve your chances of avoiding diabetes and heart disease.

Aerobic Exercise

This can include any type of activity that gets your heart rate elevated and improves your circulation by dilating and enlarging your arteries and veins. Running, skipping rope, basketball, tennis, swimming, or exercise classes are all good examples of aerobic activities that can improve your stamina and breathing. They also improve detoxification because as your circulation improves during activity, you'll maintain the same improved circulation at rest, when the detoxification process really occurs.

If you are currently very toxic, it may be difficult to exercise aggressively: increased circulation can stir up toxins that the body is having difficulty managing. So it is important to adjust your exercise intensity to your situation. You may want to follow the 30-day detox and then begin an exercise program.

Hot Water Followed by Cold Water Plunge

This protocol allows the body to rapidly transition from having dilated (open) blood vessels to constricted (closed down) blood vessels. During this transition a number of things happen: Your body releases a surge of adrenaline and endorphins, so you get an amazing rush, feeling completely awake and alive. You are also stimulating your circulation and lymphatics to rapidly push blood back to your core for improved processing and detoxification. This technique should only be done if you have a strong heart and a strong constitution. Please check with your health care provider before trying this.

Soak in a Jacuzzi or hot tub for five to ten minutes. Then dunk yourself in a tub of cold water for about thirty seconds. This can be repeated three times for maximum effect. As an alternative, you can do this in your shower at home by rapidly turning the temperature of the water from hot to cold. Try not to jump out of your shower when you do: please don't hurt yourself in the name of detoxification!

When you begin the 30-day detox diet, you will balance your blood sugar, lower your exposure to heavy metals, and take the first step to making a positive long-term lifestyle modification that can help you to reverse heart disease and diabetes, two devastating conditions. If you have already been diagnosed with either of these diseases, or with metabolic syndrome, work with your doctor as you go through this detox. You may be able to reduce your need for prescription medications if you learn to live with a cleaner, healthier diet.

Chapter 11
Correcting Hormone Imbalances

To understand how our hormones can become imbalanced, it is necessary to first understand how normal development should proceed. Sex hormones begin to affect our health as early as during fetal development. A male fetus has an XY chromosome makeup. The Y chromosome guides testicular development and testosterone production, which is necessary for male genital growth. Without testosterone, a female fetus develops. Female fetuses have an XX chromosome pattern, which allows the mother's estrogen and progesterone to guide the development of female sex characteristics, like the ovaries and uterus.

The endocrine system, which controls hormone production, is exceptionally sensitive to toxins, especially insecticides, pesticides, dioxins, phthalates, parabens, and bisphenol A. These toxins are commonly referred to as "endocrine disruptors" because they disturb the normal functioning of the endocrine system, which leads to hormone imbalances in both men and women.

These imbalances can affect us at every stage of life. We all know that what a mother consumes during pregnancy will affect the growing baby. However, it is not well known that the placenta is actually a major route of detoxification for the mother. When the mother is exposed to toxins, the same toxins are delivered directly to the baby when it is in its most vulnerable stage. The chemicals that a pregnant mother encounters have the ability to affect the sexual development of her child. These toxins act like extra doses of estrogen and can literally transform a male fetus into a female. After birth, some chemicals continue to be transferred from mother to baby through breast milk. While breast milk remains the best food for babies because of its immunological, nutritional, and psychological benefits, it is often polluted. Some of the chemicals we receive from our mothers in utero and through breast-feeding remain with us for years, affecting, or even determining, our body burden.

Endocrine disruptors are also linked to premature development of primary and secondary sexual characteristics in adolescent children. Later exposure to these chemicals can cause female and male infertility, early onset of menopause and its male equivalent andropause, and sex-hormone-related cancers, such as breast cancer and prostate cancer.

Beginning in adolescence, the sex hormone estrogen plays the predominant role in a woman's life. Estrogen is necessary for developing a female child into a woman through the stimulation of estrogen-sensitive tissue in the breasts, hips, and genitals. Women produce estrogen from the ovaries beginning around the age of twelve, when girls start to have their menstrual cycle. Estrogen and progesterone continue to be produced until menstruation ceases, typically between the ages of forty-five and fifty-five. Lack of hormone production and end of menstruation are the hallmarks of menopause, which occurs with the associated symptoms of hot flashes, night sweats, decreased libido, increased weight gain, mood swings, and overall dryness.

Men have a much less complex hormonal cycle. Around the age of twelve, boys will start producing testosterone from the testicles. Over the next six years, testosterone will stimulate the development of male sex characteristics, including increased musculature, growth in height and weight, genital hair, as well as enlarged testicles and penis. Testosterone peaks in production when a man reaches his early twenties, after which levels slowly decline. By the age of fifty-five, the levels of testosterone are about half of what they once were. Testosterone is known to be an anabolic hormone, which means it helps improve metabolism and muscle mass. As testosterone levels decline, so does metabolism and muscle mass. Older men experience their own type of menopause, called andropause, which leaves them feeling frail, gaining weight, and experiencing a decrease in libido.

If you are suffering from some of the symptoms listed in the hormone section of the detox questionnaire, you may be experiencing a hormone imbalance caused by inappropriate and inadvertent exposure to xenoestrogens. After reviewing this list, you may want to consider the detox diet as a way to help you eliminate sources of additional exposure, which will help to lower your body burden and possibly bring your hormone levels into better balance. You will also need to make more conscientious decisions when purchasing products that contain endocrine disruptors.

Insecticides and Pesticides Affect Sexual Health

The insecticides and pesticides that have estrogen-like effects are used to disrupt the fertility and growth cycle of insects and pests. Every time you go out to zap wasps with insecticide spray, you are using chemicals that affect insect and human hormones. The targets of these chemicals include mites, mosquitoes, gnats, wasps, yellow jackets, and other insects. Research suggests that less than 1 percent of the pesticides and insecticides reach their target. The rest is dispersed into the atmosphere, contaminating water, landing on non-organically grown vegetables, or being consumed by animals as part of their feed.

The insecticides and pesticides that have been created to target the endocrine system of pests also affect us. As we get exposed to these chemicals, they can interact and artificially stimulate estrogen receptors in both men and women. This leads to an excess burden of estrogen stimulation in our bodies, causing a hormonal imbalance and its associated symptoms and conditions.

TAKING CONTROL OF FETAL DEVELOPMENT

Toxic exposure in developing fetuses and breast-feeding infants is part of the reason that some doctors believe there is such a drastic increase in reported cases of autism (which now affects one in one hundred children when just two years ago it was one in one hundred and fifty), attention deficit disorder, attention deficit hyperactivity disorder (which currently affects one in sixteen children), and allergies (which affects one in four). These statistics are staggering. Fortunately, there are programs for preconception detoxification that can help detect and treat women who are concerned about their body burden.

Focus on Infertility

According to the Centers for Disease Control and Prevention in the United States roughly 12 percent of women between the ages of fifteen and forty-four have impaired fertility. This level has been increasing over the last fifty years. There are a number of theories about why we have higher infertility rates, which involve factors such as delay in the age that people are starting to have families and increased stress on families from having two parents in the workforce.

Another, more sinister, cause of infertility suggested by some researchers is exposure to xenoestrogens, which have been linked to irregular menstrual cycles and poor ovulatory cycles in women and low sperm counts in men. If you are struggling with infertility, work with your health care provider to determine the underlying cause. If no clear medical cause is determined, you may want to consider following the 30-day detox diet, which will help lower your body burden by restricting your intake to organic foods that are less likely to have xenoestrogens. You can also make better product choices, as discussed in chapter 4, to eliminate xenoestrogens from your life. The goal of this approach is to give your hormones a chance to become better balanced and thereby resume the normal fertility cycle.

Hormones and Foods

Hormones are often unnecessarily added to our lives. Aside from landing on fruits and vegetables that end up on our dinner plates and in our wine glasses, hormones are injected into livestock to make them produce more milk or to get bigger faster. These excess hormones are stored in the animals' tissue and fat. We are exposed to them when we eat nonorganic meat or drink nonorganic milk or wine. Even though we only get exposed to a low level each time, over time they build up because they are fat soluble and get stored in our body fat.

Toxic Amounts of Sugar Cause Hormone Imbalance

Toxic amounts of sugar will not only lead to heart disease and diabetes, they are also linked to hormone imbalance. Polycystic ovary syndrome (PCOS) is one of the most common female endocrine disorders, affecting up to 10 percent of women between the ages of twelve and forty-five, and is thought to be a leading cause of female infertility. The symptoms include irregular menstrual periods, loss of menstrual cycle, weight gain, and excessive hair growth. All of these symptoms are related to a typical underlying cause: insulin resistance—the same culprit that links heart disease and diabetes.

In PCOS, the toxic effects of simple sugars cause excess insulin to be excreted, which in turn causes weight gain and excess fat accumulation. Excess insulin then causes more testosterone to be released, which leads to excess hair growth. In the body's fat cells, the hormone testosterone gets converted into estrogens in a process called aromatization. This process leads to an excess amount of estrogens, which together with testosterone cause further symptoms.

In men, toxic sugar levels can cause excessive insulin release and fat accumulation, and transform testosterone into estrogen. This can lead to symptoms like enlarged breast tissue, irritability, and moodiness as well as prostate enlargement. The good news is that all of these symptoms can be easily managed by controlling blood-sugar levels, which happens naturally on the detox diet.

Molly Overcame Cancer, Then Had to Deal with Toxins

Molly came to my office looking for ideas on how to improve her post-chemotherapy symptoms. At forty-nine years old, Molly was in a good state of health after she was diagnosed and successfully treated for ovarian cancer. However, the hysterectomy she underwent after her diagnosis made her feel like her life changed for the worse. Molly told me that she always felt very fatigued. She noticed that her memory was worse. She couldn't lose weight. She was having digestive gas and bloating. She was stiff in her muscles and joints, especially her knees, and was experiencing many of the symptoms of hormone imbalance, including hot flashes, night sweats, and difficulty sleeping. Her sex drive was shot, and she had vaginal dryness. Molly had also developed fatty liver, a condition in which the liver literally gets deposited with fat, which in her case likely occurred because of the toxic effect of chemotherapy on her liver during her treatment protocol. On her detox questionnaire she scored 102 (the goal is 14 or lower). Her weight was 154 pounds.

Molly wanted to reverse many of these issues. Normally, I would prescribe bioidentical hormones for this type of patient. Yet this course of treatment was not right for Molly: because of her bout with ovarian cancer, which is an estrogen-sensitive cancer, we couldn't give her bioidentical hormone replacement therapy for fear of stimulating the growth of any remaining cancer cells.

I ordered some nutritional blood tests to see if there were any imbalances and also started her on the detox diet. I explained that the detox diet would be a good way for her body to have an opportunity to heal itself and to avoid sugar and additional xenoestrogens that might be contributing to her symptoms. While I couldn't restore her hormone function, I could help her feel more comfortable.

A month later, Molly returned to my office for her first follow-up appointment, and she said that she felt "amazing." She explained that she had 50 percent fewer hot flashes, improved energy, no digestive symptoms, no reflux, no headaches, no muscle aches, and no joint aches. She felt like her sleep had improved. She stopped drinking coffee, which she thought she would never be able to do. Her questionnaire score dropped from 102 to 20 and her weight dropped from 154 pounds to 149.

Molly's health dramatically worsened after she went through her cancer treatment, but many of her issues resolved after she followed the 30-day detox diet program, even without the use of hormone therapies. During the cancer treatment, two major things happened. First, when she had a hysterectomy and had her ovaries removed, she immediately went into menopause. While this helped her decrease the risk of cancer cell re-growth, it caused a complete disruption in her normal hormone balance. Remember, the body loves to stay in balance, and when there's an abrupt shift like this, the body's sex hormones are thrown completely out of balance. It's like taking a person who loves to be on land and sticking them on a boat in the middle of a terrible thunderstorm, even if the boat will save their life.

The chemotherapy also caused a tremendous shift in Molly's ability to heal. Chemotherapy is not only poisonous to cancer cells but also poisonous to all other cells in the body. The liver tries its best to detoxify the chemotherapy as well as it can, but chemotherapy is really a battle between the cancer cells and the cancer-cell poison. The detoxification restored better liver functionality so that Molly could lower her overall body burden. Ultimately, this made the sex hormones that she did have work more efficiently as they became more balanced.

Prostate Cancer and Toxins

For years doctors have thought that high levels of testosterone increased the risk of developing prostate cancer. Treatments were created to lower the testosterone levels of patients diagnosed with prostate cancer. Testosterone-suppressive therapies, and even castration, were treatment methods used in an attempt to control the progression of this disease. However, we now know that the reverse is true: men with low testosterone levels are more likely to have prostate cancer.

Recently, our ability to diagnose prostate cancer has become more successful. Men have been found to have evidence of prostate cancer at much earlier stages, which makes surgical treatments more effective. However, one of the truisms of medicine is that if a man lives long enough he has a 100 percent chance of developing prostate cancer. That's why many men are increasingly looking for preventative steps they can take to lower their risk of developing prostate cancer. The most recent theory on why prostate cancer develops represents a controversial paradigm shift in medical thinking. A 2010 article in the *European Journal of Cancer Prevention* points to exposure to xenoestrogens as a major risk factor in developing prostate cancer. By following the detox diet and understanding the sources of xenoestrogen exposure, you may be able to decrease your chance of developing prostate cancer.

Eric Increased His Testosterone Naturally

Eric is a forty-eight-year-old male who was in a good state of health but found that he was putting on weight because of eating large portions of food under stressful work conditions. He was craving salty foods and sugar, and was having achy muscles and joints when he came to see me. However, he was most specifically concerned because his wife felt his libido was substantially lower, a symptom he blamed on work-related stress.

Eric has three children, and he said that he had a healthy, loving marriage. In fact, it was his wife's idea that he come to see me to address his hormone symptoms. When we reviewed his symptoms, we found that his detox questionnaire score was 54 (the goal is 14 or under), and his weight was 255 pounds. Eric's wife already knew about the detox diet, and she wanted me to help guide Eric through the process. We decided that we would do some blood tests on his first visit, to check his testosterone levels, and we started the detox diet right away.

A month later, Eric returned to the office for his follow-up visit. He reported that work was still stressful, but he could handle his workload more easily. Overall, he felt more stable while he was on the detox diet. He noticed increased energy and weight loss, and he felt like his libido was returning.

He retook the questionnaire, and his score dropped from 54 to 22. We took a look at his hormone levels and saw that his testosterone level, which should be between 600 and 1,000, was 177. Anything under 300 is considered very low. We discussed whether he should consider testosterone therapy to help improve his levels and potentially improve his symptoms. Eric decided to try to do it the natural way instead and see if there was any way to bring his levels up without using hormones. So he decided to continue the detox diet for another two months, and then to follow up with another hormone check and office visit.

Eric came back two months later, this time reporting that his energy was even better, and he was definitely feeling less stressed at work. He also said that his libido was improving quite a bit. And his wife was also quite happy because she was more attracted to her husband now that he was losing so much weight. We rechecked his hormone levels and found that his testosterone had gone up to 380 from following the detox diet for three months.

What's interesting in this story is that Eric's hormone levels improved as he was going through the detoxification program. In this instance, Eric's stress at work was the tipping point. When a person is under stress, cortisol levels increase. Cortisol is considered a stress hormone, and it actually suppresses testosterone. Cortisol is also the hormone that causes stubborn belly fat to accumulate. Yet because the detox diet takes stress off the body, allowing it to heal itself, cortisol decreases and, as a consequence, testosterone levels are able to go back to where they should be.

Improving Endocrine Function and Hormone Balance with Meditation

The act of mindful meditation, or even repetitive routines, allows us not only to balance stress but also our thyroid, sex, and adrenal hormones. During the meditative state, our body enters into the rest-and-relaxation-dominant part of our autonomic nervous system function, which is called the parasympathetic nervous system. During the time of parasympathetic nervous system function, our body has a chance to recharge and heal itself in many ways, including healing the endocrine glands, which produce hormones that can improve detoxification (e.g., DHEA, testosterone, and thyroid hormone) and hormones that slow down detoxification (e.g., cortisol and adrenaline). When these hormones are properly balanced our body is able to perform detoxification functions effectively.

You can enter into a meditative state during seated meditation or while performing breathing exercises or doing tai chi, yoga, martial arts, or even something as mundane as needlework. The goal is to get the mind to become peaceful and relaxed, and to turn the focus away from the stress of day-to-day activities. Meditation can take as little as ten minutes and needs to be done regularly—ideally, every day.

Now that you understand how toxins affect specific systems within the body, you should be ready to begin your own detoxification. As you read on, you'll learn how to tailor your meal plan and your own detox to address many of these specific issues. The next chapter introduces the detox diet. You'll find that it's easier than you ever thought to eliminate environmental toxins to lose weight, increase energy, and reverse illness.

Part III
The 30-Day Detox

Chapter 12
Get Ready to Detox

Our body works like a car. We require food as an energy source, much like a car requires fuel. The more nutritious the food, or the cleaner the fuel, the better our body will work. And the body, like a car, has some self-cleaning capacities. When your car is running, the outside air and debris in the oil are filtered before they reach the engine. But like your body, a car still accumulates debris and soot in the fuel lines. That's why regular oil changes and scheduled tune-ups are recommended for the optimal performance of your vehicle. Without them, you'll find that your car's fuel efficiency will decrease over time.

The detox you are about to begin works in much the same way. You are going to change the food you eat to increase your performance. You'll be giving yourself a tune-up by giving your body an opportunity to heal itself. You'll accomplish this by focusing on the cleanest food options and selecting nutrients that will optimize your body's detoxification systems. By doing so, you're making sure that your body can continue to run smoothly and efficiently. You'll finally get rid of the toxins, chemicals, and pollutants that have been clogging your system and weighing down your health. And afterward, you'll feel significantly better.

Dr. Morrison's Detoxification Strategy

Recently, detox diets have crossed into the mainstream thanks to celebrity endorsements and marketing campaigns that suggest they lead to quick-and-easy weight loss. Some of these programs want you to fast or drink some concoction that tastes terrible and can potentially make you sick. I don't believe that either of those strategies is really a good long-term solution. First, when you fast the body is deprived of nutrition, which means there is a much higher chance that you'll regain all the weight lost once the fast is completed. Even worse, the weight lost generally consists of a significant amount of muscle rather than just fat. This is because when you fast, the liver cannibalizes muscle stores in order to maintain the adequate level of amino acids necessary to effectively drive your detoxification enzymes. A fast puts a great deal of stress on your liver, which requires certain vitamins, minerals, antioxidants, and amino acids to facilitate the detoxification processes.

I've devised a way for you to lose weight, think clearer, and feel better than you have felt in a long time. This plan will not only give you the benefits of rapid weight loss; it will also begin the transition to living a completely healthier life. This program is designed to support all the organs involved in detoxification—the liver, kidney, lungs, lymphatic system, colon, and skin—by providing the most effective foods and nutrients. Once you provide your body with the nutritional building blocks needed to heal it, it will do the rest of the work for you.

My detox diet will help you achieve great results because it combines two critical detoxification strategies: an elimination-diet meal plan (described in the next chapter) along with a nutrient-dense detox protein shake and supportive supplemental nutrients. The meal plan provides clear guidelines for how to eat a clean diet free of chemicals, toxins, and foods that may be causing weight gain and physical symptoms. Just like taking that stone out of your shoe, eliminating certain foods from your diet gives your body the chance to heal from the irritation they are causing. Without them, your body will function at a higher level, and you will have less illness and generally feel better.

The Detox Shake

I hope that you will enjoy the simplicity of using the shake as a meal replacement. The shake helps keep you feeling full and satisfied, while helping you to maintain lean body mass. My patients tell me that after the first week they want to stay on the detox shake because it tastes good and, as a consequence, helps them to easily transition to long-term healthy lifestyle habits.

When you remove processed foods, especially those that may be causing inflammation, you allow your body a chance to rest and then heal itself. And when you eliminate toxins, chemicals, and foods you might be sensitive to from your diet, your cells will become healthy and will be able to function properly again. By using the shake as a meal replacement along with the meal plan, you are doing three things at once: first, you are eliminating possible food allergies and sensitivities that are causing inflammation; second, you are eliminating the toxins and chemicals in foods that are making you sick; and third, you are adding nutrient-rich foods that give your body the support it needs to cleanse itself. The plan succeeds because it does all three of these things together.

The protein-rich detox shake is easy to make; the recipe is in the next chapter. You will be using the shake as a meal replacement twice a day. Generally, people like to have it for breakfast and lunch. However, if you are the type of person that likes to eat a bigger lunch and a smaller dinner, or if you have to eat out frequently for lunch, you can have the shake for dinner.

The shake you'll be making must contain essential amino acids that support detoxification, and in the next chapter I will show you how to choose the best protein powder sources. The term "essential amino acid" is used to describe any amino acid that your body cannot synthesize on its own and that must be derived from diet. The animal proteins found in meat, chicken, and fish have all essential amino acids, while vegetable sources like rice, soy, and beans do not. The goal is to find a protein powder that uses a vegetable protein source with the essential amino acids added.

If you do not have all the essential amino acids because your diet is deficient in protein or the correct essential amino acids, your body will either start to cannibalize protein stored in your muscle or it will not carry out the detox process completely and your symptoms could get worse.

The detox shake also supplies the vitamins, minerals, medium-chain triglycerides (MCTs), and antioxidants that are important building blocks necessary to improve liver detoxification, which happens in two distinct phases. During phase one, the liver makes fat-soluble toxins temporarily reactive and capable of being turned into water-soluble compounds, which is what occurs in phase two, so they can be safely eliminated out of the body. If there are not enough nutrients for phase two to work properly, the reactive toxins produced in phase one begin to build up in the body and can actually cause worse toxicity than the original toxin. Vitamins such as A, D, E as well as the B vitamins, along with the minerals calcium, magnesium, zinc, copper, and selenium, all assist the liver's detoxification process. Antioxidants such as the catechins from decaffeinated green tea are like the janitors of detoxification: they help to mop up free radicals that are created during the intermediate step between the two phases of detoxification. Amino acids such as taurine, L-glutathione, and N-acetylcysteine (NAC) are the building blocks of the second phase of the liver's detoxification process, available to help the body manufacture different proteins and enzymes as needed to manage the detoxification load. Medium-chain triglycerides are good fats that actually help to improve metabolism and weight loss.

The Clinical Paper

A few years ago, I realized that there were many studies that showed either the effectiveness of detoxification, or the effectiveness of weight-loss diets, but none that showed both. The primary objective of my clinical study and the resulting paper was to examine what a detox diet with meal replacement would do to symptoms of toxicity and weight loss.

We started the study by reviewing the charts of a group of thirty-one new patients who came to my practice looking for relief of physical symptoms related to toxins, weight loss, or both. Each person began, just as you have, by taking the detox questionnaire. We recorded their scores on a scale similar to the one that you have used. We also performed a physical exam that measured their current weight and height, and performed appropriate blood work to look for any possible underlying causes of the symptoms they listed in their questionnaire responses. Then they began the detoxification process.

Each participant began with a 30-day supply of the protein shake, similar to what you will be using, along with instructions on when to have the shake (i.e., for breakfast and lunch) and meal suggestions for dinner and snacks. We then asked them to follow this plan for four weeks and to come back to report on their progress.

After thirty days, the patients returned to my office for a follow-up visit to repeat the questionnaire and recheck their weight. All participants successfully completed the plan. Before and after changes in the detoxification questionnaire and subjects' weights were calculated and compared.

We were able to show a significant degree of weight loss in patients following the detox diet. The subjects lost an average of 8.9 pounds after four weeks, which compared favorably with conventional weight-loss plans: people on the Atkins diet averaged losing 9.7 pounds; Weight Watchers, 6.3 pounds; and Slim-Fast, 5.9 pounds. Given these results, we demonstrated that my detox plan is a reasonable alternative to both high-protein diets and conventional diets in terms of weight loss. As a bonus, my plan can also be used by vegans looking to lose weight.

We also monitored symptoms related to toxins. During the full five weeks of the study, all the participants were able to clearly discern that their symptoms had improved, across all categories. More important, the results were statistically significant for both weight-loss and improved-symptom scores, which means that the results were unlikely to have occurred by chance. The overall total detox score declined an average of 66.3 percent across subjects. These results compare favorably with symptoms scores in other detox studies using the same questionnaire, showing improvement of 47 percent at one week and 52 percent at ten weeks. There was no significant increase in symptoms while adhering to the detox diet. These results showed that my detox diet was useful for patients interested in losing weight and improving how they feel.

What's more, no relationship was found between the amount of weight lost and the change in detoxification scores, which is important for people who would like to participate in a detox diet but do not want to lose weight. However, I believe that people successfully lose weight on this plan because of the unique combination of the elimination diet and the low calories and high nutrient values of the foods they continue to eat.

What You Can Expect from Your Detox

My clinical experience shows that benefits are experienced within four weeks of following the program, although many of my patients start feeling better after the first week. Signs that the detox is working include a noticeable increase in energy, a general feeling of lightness, and the dissipation of many symptoms and conditions that were occurring because of your exposures to toxins and chemicals, and sensitivities to foods, in your diet. By implementing this program, you will accomplish the following:

- **Lose weight:** As you remove the sources of toxin exposure from your body, you will generally find a rapid loss of water weight and a slow and steady loss in body fat.
- **Have more energy:** As your organs, blood, and cells heal themselves they begin to function better, and you will notice that you have more energy. If the damage to your tissue is mild, you will

notice your energy return quickly; however, if the damage to your tissues is more significant, you may find that your energy takes longer to return.

- **Develop an improved sense of well-being:** When your body heals itself, you will find that you also improve in mood and spirit.
- **Create a new healthy lifestyle:** Once you realize how good you can feel, you won't want to return to the old habits that created your symptoms. You will find that you want to maintain many of the new healthy habits you have learned during this process.

Experiencing a True Detoxification

When you first start the detox diet, it's important to recognize that people generally crave the foods that they're allergic to. So if you find that you crave sugar or bread or sweets, then you're in good company because many people do. During the first three to five days, a real withdrawal process can occur. You may notice that your energy is lower, and you may temporarily feel weaker or less energetic.

This doesn't mean that you need to make any changes or increase your calories. It just means that you have to get through a transition from a toxic diet to a clean one. Generally, after five to seven days the sun starts to come out, and you'll start thinking more clearly and notice an increase in your energy.

If after seven days your energy level is not increasing, then you may need to speak with your health care provider to determine if there is a more serious underlying issue that needs to be addressed, such as a thyroid problem, a hormone imbalance, or some other serious health concern or condition that needs to be followed closely. If this is the case, you may be able to continue the detox, but you likely will need to modify it by specifically adding more of the allowable carbohydrates listed in chapter 13.

For some people, I've found, it takes a full two weeks before they begin to notice a significant change in their health. This usually has to do with their level of toxicity. If your total score on the questionnaire was above 50, you may need to be prepared for a slower detox process. That being said, in my chart review I found that some of my greatest successes occurred in patients with scores greater than 50. And some of those patients had symptom improvement in as little as one week. Everyone is different, and just remember that if you find that your detox is not going well you can always stop and speak with your health care provider about your concerns. Sometimes it just takes longer for your immune system to bounce back or for your metabolism to increase.

> **DO NOT START THIS PROGRAM IF YOU ARE**
> - Pregnant or nursing
> - Under the age of eighteen
> - Or if you have a serious illness for which your health care provider determines a weight-loss program would be contraindicated

The 30-Day Detox

The 30-day plan is geared for weight loss as well as detoxification. Every day you'll have a shake for breakfast, a snack of seasonal fruit between breakfast and lunch, a lunch of a shake and a salad, and a second snack of raw or cooked vegetables between lunch and dinner. For dinner, you'll have a meal with lean protein and vegetables. The complete diet and meal plans are outlined in the next chapter.

On the 30-day plan, you will eat about sixty grams of protein a day, which is enough to maintain muscle mass. The diet is not carbohydrate restricted, but the carbohydrates come from vegetables and the protein shake. All in all, you'll be eating roughly 1,000 to 1,200 calories a day, but don't let that scare you. I've found that my patients feel very satisfied during the thirty days; they're not hungry and they recognize that they can survive quite easily. After the initial transition period, their sugar cravings go away, and they no longer feel hungry after meals. Even though we encourage people to have snacks between breakfast and lunch, like an apple or a pear or berries, many of my patients find that the breakfast shake will hold them until lunchtime.

If you are not looking for weight loss, you will be able to add more starch and vegetables to the eating plan. In this case, you can increase your caloric intake to at least 1,500 calories per day. However, a lighter caloric load does help with the detoxification process. The fewer calories there are to digest means the better the body is able to metabolize and process toxins out of the body.

Supplements Everyone Should Take During the 30-Day Detox

In a perfect world, we would be able to get all the nutrients we need from the food we eat. However, this is not always possible. As we discussed in chapter 3, changes in modern farming have created nutritionally depleted foods. So even when you follow a diet that is high in organic fruits and vegetables, like in the 30-day detox program, you are still only getting a fraction of the nutrients these foods should contain. I have found that the best way to make sure you get the recommended daily allowance of vitamins and minerals is through nutrient supplements, such as a general multivitamin.

You don't need to take a high-potency multivitamin, which has ingredients at doses hundreds or thousands of times more potent than the recommended daily allowance, because many of the nutrients they contain can be derived from following this diet. There may also be some overlap if you choose to take other supplements for more-specific needs. For these reasons, I like the Daily Pack from Daily Benefit (one packet daily with breakfast) or the Basic Detox Nutrients from Thorne Research (three capsules daily with breakfast).

The key ingredients that your multivitamin should include are:

- Green tea extract (300 mg, 50 percent EGCG): a powerful antioxidant
- Fish oil (1,000 mg daily): high in omega-3 fatty acids

- Probiotic (at least 1 billion cfu): replaces the good bacteria that chlorinated drinking water kills
- Vitamin C (1,000 mg): powerful antioxidant and helps with connective-tissue repair

A second supplement I always recommend is yerba maté, which is made from the leaves of a tree native to the highlands of Brazil, Paraguay, and Argentina. This evergreen, a member of the holly family, produces leaves that when dried are used to create a healthful drink consumed by millions of South Americans as an alternative to coffee. It is claimed that yerba maté has the ability to provide energy without causing nervousness or the jitters that can be associated with coffee. Many use this as an alternative to green tea because of its high levels of antioxidants.

You can purchase yerba maté as a supplement or as a tea. If you do not enjoy the taste and would still like to get the health benefits, I recommend the product Tea Energy from Daily Benefit (two capsules in the morning with food). This product is a great way to overcome your coffee addiction, without the headaches.

I also recommend that you take Svetol, a decaffeinated green-coffee-bean-extract supplement that helps to improve fat burning and allows the liver to better process fat and carbohydrates. To get the correct amount of Svetol in supplement form (200 mg), I recommend the Diet Formula from Daily Benefit (two capsules twice daily for a month, and then two capsules daily until your have achieved your weight-loss goals).

Finally, I recommend that everyone take vitamin D_3 (cholecalciferol). Vitamin D is mandatory for proper calcium absorption from the digestive tract and for proper bone mineralization. As we get older, a vitamin D deficiency can lead to a loss in bone density, causing osteoporosis. Low levels of vitamin D have also been found to cause a number of other problems: Pregnant mothers with low vitamin D are more likely to have children that develop type 1 diabetes. Low vitamin D in adulthood is associated with an increased susceptibility to multiple sclerosis. People with low vitamin D tend to have low moods, especially seasonal affective disorder (described as low mood during the winter), and are more likely to have fibromyalgia, be susceptible to the flu, and are even more likely to get cancer.

Vitamin D is the only vitamin that the body manufactures from sunlight (UVB rays). Spending about ten minutes in the sun between the hours of 10:00 a.m. and 2:00 p.m. during the summer without sunscreen provides over 5,000 IU of vitamin D. However, most of us spend a great deal of time indoors and/or have become zealous about wearing sunscreen while we are in the sun (for good reason: avoiding skin cancer). While the benefits of sunscreen are valid, you cannot make vitamin D while you wear it: the UVB rays are blocked from hitting the skin. And if you live in an area with four seasons, you can't make enough vitamin D from the sun during the fall and winter months. The general rule is that if your shadow is longer that you are tall, then you aren't making vitamin D, because the sun is not high enough in the sky to provide the correct UVB wavelength. Because of these factors, we are all becoming vitamin D deficient.

You can ask your doctor to check your 25-OH vitamin D levels. They should fall between 50 and 100. It's also possible to have too much vitamin D, so I recommend a daily vitamin D_3 supplement of 1,000–5,000 IU, taken with food.

The 10-Day Seasonal Detox

The 10-day plan offers the same gentle detoxification as the 30-day plan and is meant to be used like a seasonal tune-up once you've finished the first thirty days. The 10-day program should be repeated at the beginning of the spring, summer, and fall (three times a year) for the best results. I don't generally recommend detoxing during the winter, because that is the time when most of your body's resources are focused on maintaining a well-functioning immune system. That being said, you absolutely can benefit your immune system and your health during the winter by focusing on the lifestyle modification recommendations that I make.

During the seasonal detoxes, you can incorporate as many seasonal, locally grown organic fruits and vegetables into your meal plan as you can find. You will be focusing on the food suggestions featured in the next chapter.

Preparing Your Meals: Cooking and Storing Options

Given everything that we learned about potentially toxic heavy metals and plastics, you must be wondering what to cook and store food in. You can make small changes to the way you cook food to avoid creating more AGEs and ingesting toxins. On the 30-day program, you'll be avoiding charred or browned foods. All proteins should be steamed, braised, poached, or baked. When you add water to the cooking process, you limit the formation of AGEs.

You can also broil or grill lean proteins at a lower heat so your fish or poultry doesn't become browned. If you do have blackened sections, you can always cut off and discard those charred parts.

Generally, try to avoid cooking your food in the following:

- **Nonstick cookware:** This can be hazardous to your health and to the environment. The nonstick coating is made from a fluoride molecule, either fluoropolymer or polytetrafluoroethylene (PTFE), which we know to be extremely toxic. If you use nonstick cooking surfaces, make sure that you do not cook on high heat, which causes the coating to vaporize, and never use metal instruments on the cooking surface, which can easily scratch the surface, making the nonstick coating even more volatile.
- **Aluminum cookware:** Aluminum can build up in the body and may cause neurodegenerative conditions like Alzheimer's disease.

Cast iron is a healthy cooking option that is great for cooking meat, is safe to use at high temperatures, and is very durable. The main downside is that it can be heavy. Stainless steel is also very good option and certainly preferable to nonstick, but make sure that there is no aluminum coming in contact with your food. Many times stainless steel has an aluminum core to make it lighter. Stainless steel is made from a combination of iron, chromium, and nickel, so if you have a nickel allergy, this may not be the right option for you.

Ceramic cookware is another good option. It is resistant to cracking, has a high heat resistance, is relatively nonstick, is lightweight, and is very nontoxic. The main drawback is that it is fragile and can break if dropped.

Most storage options involve some type of plastic or glassware. I highly recommend that you invest in glass food-storage containers because they have no susceptibility to leach toxic chemicals into foods. Their main drawback is that they can be heavy and they can break when dropped.

Plastic storage containers are another option. These are safe as long as the plastic is not heated, which could occur if they are used to reheat food or if hot food is placed directly into them without first having an opportunity to cool. Also, plastic containers tend to absorb smells and may not be able to withstand the heat from dishwashers.

WRAPPING FOOD

I generally recommend that you avoid using aluminum foil that touches your food. Small amounts of aluminum exposure can over time lead not only to Alzheimer's-like symptoms but also to aching muscles and softer bones (think osteoporosis). Plastic wrap is not a better option. The plastic leaches into the food with heat and leaves residues in the food, which when consumed act as endocrine disruptors. A better option is old-fashioned, natural, unbleached wax paper. Natural wax is safe and nontoxic. Wax paper can be used to store food and line trays for baking. The main drawback is that it can burn, so be careful about using it in the oven.

Pass on the Microwave

Microwave cooking should be avoided. Even though microwave ovens have created a great deal of time savings in preparing food, it is at a cost both to the quality of our food and to our health. Basically, microwaving makes the food less valuable to your cells. The microwave oven creates an intensely high heat in the very center of food. This heat is so high that it can denature or destroy normal protein structure and deactivate vitamins, minerals, and enzymes in the food. This type of heat is very different from cooking in the oven and on the stovetop, where food is heated slowly and evenly.

Also, microwaves can leak from the oven during food preparation and affect anything within close proximity of the unit. Even though the microwave oven seems self-contained, standing too close to one that is on can cause you to receive small amounts of radiation. So if you do use a microwave oven, don't stick your face up against the glass to see how far your food has come along, because you may end up getting exposed to microwaves.

Quick Tips for Eating Out

Here are some of my best tips for staying on the program even when you have to eat out of your home, and in restaurants:

1. Choose your restaurant wisely: Before you go out, do a little home-work and learn about the menu ahead of time. Many restaurants post their menus online, and if they don't, you can call the restaurant to find out what they are serving. I would recommend that you decide what you are going to eat before you get there; this way you won't be tempted by what everyone else is eating.
2. Banish the bread basket: As soon as you sit down for dinner, make a pact with your dinner guests to send the bread basket back to the

kitchen before it gets placed on the table. Once that bread is on the table, it is very difficult for even the most committed detoxers to avoid.

3. Stick to appetizers and side dishes: Not only will you have a great selection, but you'll save money as well. You can easily order a large mesclun salad with shrimp, 100 percent crabmeat, or fish, and a side of beets or sautéed spinach and feel completely satisfied.

4. Save dessert for when you deserve it: You have made a commitment to follow this plan for thirty days. If you really want to savor a dessert, wait until you have met your goal, and then give yourself a little prize for your hard work.

5. Follow the Morrison method of ordering:
   • Choose a large salad dressed with olive oil and lemon juice
   • Choose a lean protein: chicken, fish, and turkey are great options
   • Choose a side dish: for example, beets, sautéed spinach, okra, or escarole
   • Drink about eight ounces of water during dinner

6. If you must have a drink with dinner, keep it clear: This means definitely do not have beer or wine while on the detox diet. Both beer and wine have too much sugar, which will invariably trigger cravings for dessert, a piece of bread, or other bad food choices. Instead have one vodka and soda or even one tequila, which are less likely to cause cravings. However, since you have been detoxing, your tolerance for alcohol will be lower because you have been consuming less alcohol, so please arrange for a designated driver.

Sleep Is Critical for Success

Because detoxification happens during rest, we must strive to get at least six to eight hours of sleep every night. We need to give our body and mind a chance to recover. When we sleep, the body is going through a short fast. This allows the cells, tissue, liver, and kidneys time to repair themselves from the stresses of the day. Additionally, our brain is recharging neurotransmitters and our body is actually healing and detoxifying itself.

If you are constantly under stress, you produce excessive amounts of fight-or-flight hormones like adrenaline, and you could have a great deal of trouble falling asleep or even staying asleep. When this happens, the body will not have the opportunity to detoxify effectively at night.

If you get less sleep on one night, try to make it up the next night. I always suggest that to ensure better sleep you should remove the television from your bedroom or turn it off by 9:00 p.m. The TV is very distracting and can easily keep a person awake much longer than they would be if it were not on. Keep your bedroom as dark as possible: when your door is closed, you should not be able to see your hand waving in front of your face. Without light, the body is able to produce the sleep hormone melatonin, which helps your body create better sleep patterns. If you work a job at night and sleep during the day, do your best to re-create a very light working environment and a pitch black sleep environment.

Last, the first thing that you should do when you wake up is go to the bathroom and eliminate urine and stool. Most people will urinate as soon as they wake up; however, I find that at least 50 percent of my patients did not make a habit of having a bowel movement in the morning. This is a sign of mild constipation. Worse, when the colon is not emptying within twelve to twenty-four hours after consuming food, the toxins in the stool have a chance to get reabsorbed and recirculated in the body.

Now that you're prepared to detox, we can discuss the meal plan.

Chapter 13
The Meal Plan

The core of the 30-day detox diet is the meal plan and food selections, which allow you to eliminate chemicals, toxins, and food sensitivities that you have been exposing yourself to. This "elimination diet" focuses on nonallergenic, nutrient-dense, seasonal, organic, locally grown foods. While eating these fruits, vegetables, and protein sources, your body will become less inflamed, and you will have fewer food cravings (especially for sugar) and fewer physical and emotional symptoms than when you started. You may also notice that you have more energy, focus, and an overall sense of well-being.

You will begin the diet by referring back to your total score in the detox questionnaire in chapter 2. Record this number directly in the book. Then record your current weight. Do not weigh yourself more than once a week on the 30-day program, because there will be some days when you gain weight and some days when you lose weight. The goal is to focus on following the overall plan and not the day-to-day fluctuations. You'll see in the end that your weight goes in the right direction. Then, when you are done with the 30-day program, you will complete the detox questionnaire again and recheck your weight.

In order to ensure that you are able to follow this plan successfully, and that your body will have the nutrients that it needs to improve your detoxification process, you'll be having two servings of the nutritious shake that has the vitamins, minerals, antioxidants, and amino acids your body will need to achieve great results. Generally, I recommend that you have the shake for breakfast and then at either lunch or dinner. The meal at which you do not have a shake should include a protein and some of the vegetables listed below.

The Detox Shake Basic Recipe

This protein detox shake can easily be mixed, shaken, or blended at home and at work. All the necessary ingredients can be purchased online or at a health food store or through my Web site (www.dailybenefit.com). Start with a nonallergenic protein source. I generally recommend using a protein powder made of brown rice, pea protein, or artichoke protein. Avoid whey-, soy-, and egg-protein powders because of the possibility for allergies. When choosing a protein powder, be sure the ingredients include all of the following essential amino acids: L-glycine, L-glutamine, DL-methionine, L-threonine, and L-lysine. Each serving should have at least fifteen grams of protein.

Besides the protein powder, you will need to mix in a soluble fiber such as ground flaxseed fiber or psyllium husk, which helps to bind toxins in the digestive tract. These fibers help to prevent re-absorption and to facilitate removal of toxins during your daily bowel movements.

You'll also be adding cinnamon, which not only makes the shake taste great but is also useful to curb sugar cravings and to maintain healthy blood-sugar levels. Finally, I recommend adding lecithin, which contains the good fat phosphatidylcholine that is thought to help improve the liver's ability to remove fat from the body and to improve the liver's and brain's ability to heal themselves. Lecithin can also help decrease the risk of gallstones. It is well known by doctors that when a patient begins a weight-loss process, if the weight loss is too rapid gallstones can sometimes form; these are called "cholesterol gallstones." They occur because the liver is taking a large burden of fat out of the body, and lecithin can help to prevent the cholesterol from getting stuck in the gallbladder.

To make the shake, use the following:

- Brown rice, pea, or artichoke protein: two scoops or at least fifteen grams of protein
- Ground flaxseed or psyllium husk fiber: one tablespoon (you may add more if you are constipated)
- Lecithin: two tablespoons
- Cinnamon: one-quarter teaspoon
- Water: eight ounces

Put all of these ingredients into a cup, blender bottle, or blender. You can stir them up, shake them, or blend them with ice cubes. Many of my patients think the shake tastes best when it's blended with ice cubes, while others like it to be thicker, so they add less water and it has a consistency more like porridge or grits than a shake. Either way, the shake is very satisfying and will keep you feeling full for hours.

Variations on the Shake

You can also add a one-half cup of organic fresh or frozen blueberries, raspberries, or strawberries to the shake to add variety, taste, and more antioxidants. Also, if you want to be really creative, we have found that adding one-half cap of almond extract, one-half cap of coffee extract, or one-half cap of vanilla extract and a teaspoon of 100 percent pure cocoa powder, or any combination of these, creates a delicious variation to the original recipe without adding a single calorie. I personally like the combination of half a capful of almond and coffee extracts, which makes the shake taste like a mochaccino.

When you purchase flavor extracts, make sure that they are 100 percent natural. I generally recommend the Frontier brand because

the extracts are organic, fair-trade certified, and alcohol free (www
.frontiercoop.com). Another brand to consider is Nature's Flavors
(www.naturesflavors.com); its extracts are 100 percent organic, alcohol
free, and kosher.

Comparing Apples and Oranges: The Detox Shake versus Real Food Choices

If you have ever dieted before, I'm sure you realize how easy it is to eat
more calories than you might suspect. And dieting is more than count-
ing calories: you need to keep track of the type of calories that are being
consumed. For example, a typical cereal or granola breakfast served
with half a cup of skim milk has approximately the same calorie count
as the detox shake; however, almost all the calories are coming from
carbohydrates. A more nutritious breakfast would include the right balance of protein, fat, and carbohydrates to keep your blood sugar stable.

Lunch and dinner can be equally dangerous in terms of calories. For
example, what appears to be a harmless chicken sandwich can be loaded
with calories from carbohydrates and fat and, worst of all, can contain
about half of your daily requirement of sodium. You need no more than
2,400 mg of sodium daily, but for people with high blood pressure the
recommendation is to have about half that amount, or 1,500 mg daily. It
is much healthier to have 3,500 mg of potassium every day, which generally comes from eating lots of vegetables and fruit.

Another acceptable option for blood-sugar control is to eat a low-
carbohydrate meal plan, which also happens to successfully help people
lose weight. According to the A TO Z Weight Loss Study, published in
the *Journal of the American Medical Association* in 2007, a lower carbohydrate intake was associated with more weight loss and more favorable
overall improvements in lowering cholesterol and blood pressure and
improving blood-sugar levels. Using the detox shake helps to ensure
that you are getting all the useful, healthy nutrition your body needs,
without excessive amounts of salt or too many carbohydrates.

Typical **Nutritional Analysis for One** Detox Shake

This analysis may change depending on the type of protein powder you use.

Total calories:	253
Fat:	10.8 g
Fat from lecithin:	9 g
Carbohydrates:	25.5 g
Dietary fiber:	3.5 g
Protein:	15.5 g
Sodium:	76 mg
Potassium:	485 mg

Nutritional Analysis for a Typical Breakfast

One-half cup Heartland Granola Cereal with skim milk (according to the Daily Plate: www.thedailyplate.com).

	½ CUP HEARTLAND GRANOLA CEREAL	½ CUP SKIM MILK	TOTAL
Total calories:	240	40	**280**
Fat:	6 g	0	**6 g**
Fat from lecithin:	N/A	N/A	**N/A**
Carbohydrates:	41 g	6 g	**47 g**
Dietary fiber:	4 g	0 g	**4 g**
Protein:	6 g	4 g	**10 g**
Sodium:	120 mg	60 mg	**180 mg**
Potassium:	200 mg	191 mg	**391 mg**

Nutritional Analysis for a Typical Lunch Option

Wawa Chicken Salad Sandwich and eight ounces of Glaceau Vitamin Water (according to the Daily Plate: www.thedailyplate.com).

	WAWA CHICKEN SALAD SANDWICH	8 OZ. GLACEAU VITAMIN WATER	TOTAL
Total calories:	527	40	567
Fat:	29 g	0	29 g
Fat from lecithin:	N/A	N/A	N/A
Carbohydrates:	41 g	9 g	50 g
Dietary fiber:	3 g	0 g	3 g
Protein:	20 g	0 g	20 g
Sodium:	908 mg	0 mg	908 mg
Potassium:	0 mg	70 mg	70 mg

The Meal Plan: Detox Does Not Mean Deprive

You will use the shake to replace breakfast and have a shake with a salad for lunch. Then you will have a sensible dinner, which you can choose from the meal plan. Each dinner focuses on lean protein and fresh grilled, steamed, or raw vegetables.

One thing you'll notice right away is that carbohydrates are limited to fruits and vegetables. When I worked with Dr. Robert Atkins, I came to recognize how carbs can adversely affect a person's health. However, Dr. Atkins and I differ on some of the details. For example, I do not advocate eating lots of red meat. This is especially important during the summer. Red meat can be very warming to the body, and during the summer the last thing anyone wants is to raise their body temperature. If you choose to eat red meat, pick lean sources and whenever possible choose 100% grass-fed instead of grain-fed beef.

Also, I do recommend eating lots of vegetables, even starchy vegetables. This means that people can snack on carrots, beets, celery, or cucumbers. Some people use avocados in their salads, as well as squash and zucchini, all of which I feel are acceptable. So when I say we avoid carbohydrates, I'm referring primarily to grains and beans. This includes avoiding brown rice, millet, lentils, and quinoa along with other "white" carbohydrates like white breads, white potatoes, and pasta. Even though brown rice, millet, lentils, and quinoa are all considered whole foods and healthy carbohydrates, we will eliminate these for a minimum of one month. This is the most important part of optimizing the weight-loss part of the meal plan. If you are not interested in losing weight, then it is acceptable to include those whole foods. However, I have found that

SUPER VEGETABLES

You will see a few vegetables repeated throughout the meal plan. For example, I love celery because it is loaded with potassium and fiber, and I have found that this tends to lower high blood pressure and helps people have daily bowel movements. Always choose organic celery: it tastes much better and has much less pesticide residue.

Carrots are thought to have a lot of sugar, but they also have a lot of fiber, which means the amount of sugar contained within the carrot is slowly absorbed and does not have an overwhelming impact on your blood sugar. Carrots are loaded with the antioxidant beta-carotene, which is needed during the interim step between phase one and two liver detoxification.

Beets are another starchy vegetable that are good to eat on this plan, because they contains lots of betaine, which is also known as trimethyl glycine (TMG) and is a great aid in liver detoxification.

when my patients avoid grains and beans for a month, they find that they feel great and do not miss them.

Acceptable Foods on the Detox Diet

For the next thirty days, you will be eating fruit in the morning and proteins and vegetables throughout the day. Fruits have a lot of sugar in them, which is why they taste great. They are a much better option than processed sweets because they also have antioxidants, vitamins, minerals, and electrolytes in the correct ratios that our body needs. However, like any type of sugar, fruit sugars are energy sources that are ready to be used immediately. If you eat fruit before noon, you will have all day to burn off the sugar that is ready for your body to use. However, if you eat fruit too late in the day, the sugar will not get burned off and you will just end up storing the extra calories as body fat.

It is also better to eat fruits as they become available in your region: when they are in season. Our world has become a global market and as a consequence we can get any food we like whenever we like it. This is not necessarily a good thing. When fruits are shipped long distances, they need to be sprayed with chemicals to slow their ripening process. Also, fruits grown outside the United States are not subject to the same pesticide laws that our farmers follow, so you may become exposed to the very unhealthy pesticides we are trying to avoid. A great resource for information about how to eat locally is the Eat Well Guide (www .eatwellguide.org).

In the spring look for fresh grapefruits, unless you are taking a prescription medication, like statins, which prohibits their use. Berries are good choices in spring or summer, as are plums, melons, papaya, and kiwi. In the fall and winter choose apples and pears.

FOODS TO ENJOY EVERY DAY	EAT FRUIT IN THE MORNING ONLY
Water: 1–2 liters	Grapefruit
Vegetables: steamed, sautéed, raw (see list below)	Kiwi
Olive oil	Berries
Lemon juice	Apples
Spices	Cherries
Green tea	Papaya
Once a day: 4–6 oz. of chicken, turkey, fish (tilapia, red snapper, fresh or canned Alaskan salmon, sardines, shrimp, catfish, blue crab), organic eggs	Melon
	Pears

Non- and mildly starchy vegetables everyone can enjoy:

- asparagus
- avocado
- beets and beet greens
- bok choy
- broccoli
- brussels sprouts
- cabbage
- cauliflower
- celery
- chicory
- collard greens
- crookneck squash
- cucumber
- dandelion
- endive
- escarole
- green/wax beans
- kale
- kohlrabi
- leeks
- mushrooms
- mustard greens

- okra
- onions
- parsley
- parsnips
- radishes
- romaine lettuce
- rutabaga
- scallions

- spinach
- sprouts
- summer squash
- Swiss chard (chard)
- turnips
- watercress
- zucchini

Sea Vegetables

If you enjoy Asian food, you'll find that sea vegetables are an absolutely great addition to your meals. If you are new to eating seaweed, do not be afraid! Seaweed salads taste great. Choose seaweed that is in as close to its natural form as possible. This means that if the seaweed salad looks fluorescent green, it probably has been processed and food colorings and additives have been added.

You can prepare seaweed at home by buying dehydrated wakame and simply soaking it in warm filtered water, then adding olive oil and a few drops of sesame oil. You can eat it straight, or add it to a salad, or have it with fish along with other vegetables like wilted spinach or broccoli rabe.

Here are some examples of types of seaweed to choose from (feel free to follow preparation instructions on the packaging, as long as they stick to the detox diet guidelines):

- arame
- dulse
- hijiki
- kelp
- laver
- nori
- wakame

Special Considerations

People who have a body mass index (BMI) below 18.5 are generally considered underweight and should not pursue further weight loss. BMI is a statistical measurement of a person's height and weight, which is just an estimate of healthy weight; it is not an exact science. Some people can have a low BMI or a high BMI and it can be normal for them.

BMI RANGES

Category	BMI Range (kg/m²)
Severely underweight	Less than 16.5
Underweight	From 16.5 to 18.4
Normal	From 18.5 to 24.9
Overweight	From 25 to 30
Obese	Greater than 30

To calculate your BMI, plug your height and weight into either of these equations: $BMI = weight (kg) / height (meters)^2$ or $BMI = weight (pounds) \times 703 / height (in)^2$.

Directions for Athletes

For our purposes, active athletes are defined as people who work out at least four days a week for thirty to forty-five minutes or more and raise their heart rate above 120 beats per minute at some point during the workout. Athletes need to add more carbohydrates to their meals and should try to get at least one gram of protein per pound of body weight, especially on the days they work out. This means that if you weigh 150 pounds, you should make sure that you are consuming at least 150 grams of protein to meet your daily requirements. If you are athletic and still trying to get a little bit leaner, then add the extra carbs at lunch and dinner only on the days when you are working out.

If your BMI is greater than 25 and you want to lose weight, and you're working out at a high-intensity level, then it's not mandatory to add more carbs. Again, just make sure that you are getting one gram of protein per pound of body weight so that you do not lose muscle mass. Finally, pay attention to your energy level. The only reason that you would add more carbs if your BMI is over 25 is if you find that your energy is dropping during workouts. Even high-intensity athletes can follow this meal plan with the low-carbohydrate recommendations as long as they're not getting weak.

Directions for Vegetarians

Vegetarians can follow this plan as well. The detox shake has fifteen grams of protein per shake, so by having two shakes a day you are meeting about half of your daily protein needs. The rest of the protein that you will be consuming can come from the vegetables you are eating. Vegetarians, however, always have more difficulty losing weight because they are used to having their protein from bean sources, like soy. So once a day include one-half to one cup of beans in your meal plan. And if you are an athlete and a vegetarian, you will also need to add more carbohydrates on the days that you exercise. The best time to add these carbs is after your workout, when your metabolism is working its hardest to burn calories.

Expand Your Options If Weight Loss Is Not a Goal

If you do not want to lose weight or if you live an active lifestyle, follow these directions: For breakfast you could have a shake with two servings of fruit, like half a grapefruit and half a cup of berries, to add more carbohydrates to your plan. At lunch have your shake with a salad that features black beans or lentils or garbanzo beans. At dinner have six ounces of protein with vegetables and add half a cup of millet, brown rice, or quinoa.

Choose these starchy vegetables to add necessary calories:

- artichoke
- carrots
- delicata squash
- pumpkin
- sweet potato (yams)
- winter squash

Foods Everyone Will Avoid

For the first thirty days, you will be avoiding tomatoes, white potatoes, eggplant, and peppers, which are nightshade vegetables. These can be inflammatory and cause joint stiffness or rashes. After the 30-day detox, you can reintroduce them, one at a time, to see if they actually do affect your health. Here are the foods and beverages to avoid:

FOODS TO AVOID	BEVERAGES TO AVOID
Bananas	Coffee
Grapes	Soda
Oranges	Alcohol
Tomatoes	
Potatoes	
Eggplants	

Peppers	
Corn	
Grains	
Milk/dairy products	
Soy	
Raw fish	

A Sample 30-Day Meal Plan

The following meal suggestions can be used as a guide for creating your own 30-day program. Feel free to choose among any of these meals. For example, you can swap dinners and lunches and snacks as you see fit and of course choose other foods from the "foods to enjoy" lists. If you decide to follow the suggestions below exactly as written, repeat the cycle three times to get through the first thirty days.

Day 1

Breakfast: detox shake

Snack: ½ grapefruit

Lunch: detox shake plus green leafy salad dressed with olive oil and lemon juice

Snack: 1 cup steamed broccoli with garlic, salt, and pepper

Dinner: large salad, 4–6 oz. of baked salmon served with steamed spinach

Day 2

Breakfast: detox shake

Snack: ½ cup blueberries or raspberries

Lunch: detox shake served with raw spinach salad with raw cauliflower

Snack: 1 large Kirby cucumber or carrot

Dinner: 2–3 eggs scrambled with 1 cup sautéed zucchini and summer squash

Day 3

Breakfast: detox shake

Snack: 1 green or yellow kiwi

Lunch: detox shake served with 2 cups roasted beets

Snack: 1 cup raw snow peas

Dinner: 4–6 oz. of baked chicken with broccoli and fresh lemon juice

Day 4

Breakfast: detox shake

Snack: 1 organic Golden Delicious apple

Lunch: detox shake served with 1 heaping cup of steamed bok choy

Snack: ½ cup raw green beans

Dinner: 4–6 oz. of dill-baked tilapia fillet with steamed spinach with garlic and lemon

Day 5

Breakfast: detox shake

Snack: ½ cup papaya cubes

Lunch: detox shake served with 1 avocado sliced over a large arugula salad

Snack: 3 stalks organic celery sticks

Dinner: large radish salad with 4–6 oz. of roast turkey with 1 cup of roasted cauliflower

Day 6

Breakfast: detox shake

Snack: ½ cup of any melon

Lunch: detox shake served with mesclun salad greens dressed with olive oil and lemon juice

Snack: 1 cup steamed asparagus spears

Dinner: 2 hard-boiled eggs served with roasted kale, mushrooms, and steamed beets

Day 7

Breakfast: detox shake

Snack: 1 organic Bosc pear

Lunch: detox shake served with endive and arugula salad

Snack: 1 cup steamed or roasted brussels sprouts

Dinner: 4–6 oz. of baked rosemary chicken with 1 heaping cup of roasted broccoli and onions

Day 8

Breakfast: detox shake

Snack: ½ cup cherries

Lunch: detox shake and large Swiss chard and mustard green salad dressed with olive oil and lemon juice

Snack: steamed broccoli with garlic, salt, and pepper

Dinner: 4–6 oz. of red snapper with steamed spinach drizzled with olive oil

Day 9

Breakfast: detox shake

Snack: ½ cup of organic strawberries

Lunch: detox shake served with endive and dandelion green salad

Snack: 3 large organic celery sticks

Dinner: 1 cup steamed shrimp with 1 cup sautéed onions and zucchini

Day 10

Breakfast: detox shake

Snack: 1 organic green apple

Lunch: detox shake served with 1 cup steamed broccoli

Snack: ½ avocado, sliced

Dinner: 4–6 oz. of poached salmon over large mixed green salad dressed with olive oil, pinch of sea salt, and pepper

Salad Dressing Suggestions

My standard salad dressing is two teaspoons olive oil to one teaspoon of apple cider vinegar (not balsamic vinegar) or lemon juice. I like this dressing because it's easy to make at home and also easy to order when you are at a restaurant.

However, I know that salads can get boring, so here are some other acceptable dressing options. For each one, whisk all ingredients together in a bowl until smooth. These dressings are great for salad greens, and you can also serve them as dips for raw veggies, or on top of rehydrated seaweed, or even as a marinade for chicken or fish.

One ingredient that may be new to you is coconut butter. I like this alternative to olive oil because of its unique taste and health value. It is made from whole coconut flesh and is considered to be a complete whole food, containing healthy fats, dietary fiber, protein, vitamins, and minerals. Coconut butter is soft above 80°F and solid at lower temperatures. You can soften coconut butter by putting the jar inside a bowl of warm water. You can get the coconut butter at most good health food stores.

Sweet Basil and Flaxseed Oil Dressing

This particular dressing is fantastic on seaweed salad, especially with the sea vegetable arame. It is one of my favorites.

4 tbs. flaxseed oil
2 tbs. coconut aminos
1 garlic clove, finely chopped
¼ tsp. onion powder
1 tsp. basil (fresh or dried)
2 tbs. coconut cider vinegar or apple cider vinegar (healthier substitutes for balsamic vinegar)
cracked pepper to taste
1 tbs. coconut butter

Refreshing Mint and Olive Dressing

This can be served on salad greens or tossed with a cucumber salad, or used as a sauce for chicken.

1 tbs. lemon juice
1 tbs. lime juice
4 tbs. extra-virgin olive oil
1 tbs. coconut butter
sea salt and cracked pepper to taste
¼ tsp. garlic powder
pinch of basil (fresh or dried)
2 tbs. fresh mint, chopped

The 3-3 Dressing

I gave this dressing this name because it contains walnut oil and flax, both of which are good sources of omega-3 fatty acids.

4 tbs. walnut oil
4 tbs. flaxseed oil
1 ½ tbs. lime juice
3 tbs. lemon juice
1 garlic clove, finely chopped
sea salt and cracked pepper to taste
¼ tsp. onion powder
2 tbs. chopped fresh parsley
2 tbs. chopped fresh cilantro
1 ½ tbs. apple cider vinegar

Basic Olive Oil Vinaigrette

The secret to this dressing is Bragg Sea Kelp Delight Seasoning, which is a mix of twenty-four herbs and spices. It can be found at health food stores. You can substitute your favorite herb or spice mix.

    4 tbs. olive oil

    2 tbs. apple cider vinegar

    ½ tsp. sea salt

    1 tsp. Bragg Sea Kelp Delight Seasoning

Spicy Flax Dressing

This one is great for salads as well as sauce over chicken. Spoon over baked chicken right before serving.

    4 tbs. flaxseed oil

    2 tbs. coconut aminos

    ¼ tsp. ground mustard seed

    ¼ tsp. ground ginger

    ¼ tsp. ground coriander

    cracked pepper

    ¼ tsp. curry powder

Drink Lots of Water

When you're following the program, make sure to drink one to two liters of filtered or spring water per day. Refer back to chapter 3 for my suggestions for water filters and the types of spring waters to choose. In general, try to drink out of glass, instead of plastic, especially if your water container is going to get heated during the day. Remember, when plastic is heated its chemical components leach into the water. Plastics are endocrine disruptors, which are known to increase the risk of cancer.

Other Acceptable Beverages

Coffee is not a great fluid source, and I recommend avoiding it as much as possible. It has sixty to one hundred milligrams of caffeine per serving and relatively few antioxidants, and it is acidic. The body detoxifies best in an alkaline environment, so when coffee is consumed, it will slow your detoxification process. Also, some people who are addicted to coffee or drink lots of it to stay awake and/or lose weight can drink as many as three to six cups daily without even realizing it. All of that artificial stimulation from caffeine, plus the acidity from the coffee, will cause them to become dehydrated and feel achy. I have had many patients tell me they can't live without coffee, only to find that after the first week on the detox diet they are feeling more energetic than they ever did, and without all the side effects. If you really just can't give up the taste of coffee, then I recommend you switch to having one espresso daily, and hold the cream and sugar.

A warm cup of tea is a better choice for taking in extra fluids because it has many other benefits. Green tea, for example, has a nice balance of antioxidants with a little bit of caffeine, about thirty milligrams per serving, and a calming amino acid called theanine. However, your tea intake should be separate from your water intake because tea is also a diuretic. When a substance causes you to lose water through the kidneys, it also causes the loss of electrolytes and minerals. Electrolytes like sodium and potassium help to maintain proper fluid balance within our cells. Minerals like magnesium are important to prevent muscle cramping.

If you must have caffeine during the day, choose unsweetened green tea. You can sweeten your tea yourself with stevia or xylitol (which is made from birch bark and sold as XyloSweet), both non-caloric sweeteners from natural sources. The other artificial sweeteners are thought to increase the risk of cancer and they affect insulin levels, which actually cause you to crave them even more.

You can also choose decaffeinated herbal teas any time of the day. Try to buy organic teas or brands made from plants grown in the United States, so they are less likely to be sprayed with chemicals or toxins.

There are many detox teas on the market, and many have merit. They contain different blends of ingredients depending on the source. The Alvita brand (www.alvita.com) has one of the largest selections of herbal teas.

Some specific teas to consider for your detox include the following:

- Dandelion tea: good for liver and kidney support
- Silymarin tea: good antioxidant for the liver
- Ginger tea: helps improve digestion and settles the stomach
- Chamomile tea: helps the whole body, especially your muscles, to relax
- Nettle tea: helps with allergy symptoms
- Lemon tea: works like a natural diuretic
- Rose hips tea: improves immune system function because it is high in vitamin C
- Lemongrass tea: helps to detoxify the lungs, calms the body, and acts like a mild natural diuretic

Juicing

Juicing is definitely worthwhile and a great way to make sure to get your full servings of fruits and vegetables in a meal. You can juice any of your snacks on the detox diet. This is an especially good option if you have poor digestive absorption, chronic infections, cancer, or some other health care problem that requires a higher level of nutrition.

Juicing extracts the most nutritious part of the vegetable or fruit and puts it into a more easily absorbable liquid form. However, juices need to be freshly prepared: the orange juice or pomegranate juice for sale at the supermarket is not the same as fresh juice. I generally prefer using a Vita-Mix juicer, since it preserves much of the fruit's or vegetable's fiber as well. However, if you have a severe medical problem and your digestive tract is having difficulty processing food, it is better to keep the fiber out and use a traditional juicer.

Of course, when you juice vegetables or fruits, always use organic produce. When drinking juice, you are consuming three to five times the amount of the vegetables or fruits than if you ate them whole. That means the potential for getting exposed to pesticides and other chemicals is three to five times greater, making the organic choice even more important.

Personalizing Your Meal Plan

You may need to modify the meal plan to address your results from the detox questionnaire as well as other symptoms or conditions you may be experiencing. There are specific foods that are enormously beneficial to the functioning of specific internal systems. For example, research has shown that beets improve liver detoxification and digestion; celery can help to lower blood pressure; cucumbers, parsley, and dandelion greens work as natural diuretics; cabbage, broccoli, kale, and brussels sprouts have a cleansing effect on the mucus membranes of the intestine and colon and can help relieve ulcers and constipation.

Group 1: Improving Neurological Function

- Choose good fats: Even though everyone has heard about the importance of omega-3 fatty acids for cardiovascular health, you may not realize that medium-chain triglycerides (MCTs) are essential for brain health. MCTs are found in coconut oil and coconut butter, and research is now suggesting that a diet high in MCTs can actually prevent progression and possibly reverse neurodegenerative conditions.
- Herbs/spices: My colleague Dr. Eric Braverman has written extensively about the benefits of using spices to improve brain chemistry. In his book *The Younger (Thinner) You Diet*, he goes into great detail about how black pepper augments brain dopamine levels or using cinnamon improves GABA levels. For a thorough review of spices for improving brain biochemistry, please see his book.

Group 2: Improving Immune Function

- **Lungs:** Many people following the detox diet notice that they are less susceptible to asthma and bronchitis. This is partially because they are avoiding dairy products, which can increase mucus formation, and they are avoiding sugar, which can weaken the immune system. If one of your goals is to improve lung function, try to eat more onions, horseradish, and garlic, which can work like natural expectorants. Also, sprinkle thyme on your vegetables or protein choices to help clear lung mucus.

- **Skin:** Many people following the detox diet notice that their skin rashes begin to clear as they avoid the irritating foods like tomato and soy. Avoiding processed foods also decreases the amount of bad fats in the diet, which allows the skin to heal itself. Eating avocados, which have lots of essential fatty acids, improves the skin, as does Alaskan salmon, which is loaded with omega-3 fatty acids.

- **Immune System:** People also notice that they have a better tolerance or are not susceptible to colds or allergies after completing one month on the detox diet. Again, avoiding sugar, dairy products, and processed foods helps take stress off the body. Berries and cherries have lots of antioxidants to improve the immune system. Also, garlic and shiitake and maitake mushrooms help your body to fight off infections.

Group 3: Improving Weight Loss and Digestion

- **Liver and the Digestive Tract:** Bitter herbs and vegetables are excellent to improve liver and gallbladder function. These foods include broccoli, broccoli rabe, brussels sprouts, cabbage, collard greens, and kale. Ginger is excellent for calming the stomach and improving digestion. Artichoke is thought to improve bile flow. Beets are great for the liver because of trimethyl glycine (TMG).

- **Kidneys:** Many of my patients tell me that within one week of start-ing the detox diet they notice significantly less fluid retention in their hands and feet. Part of the reason for this is that they are avoiding processed foods that have lots of salt. Another reason is that they are eating foods that work like natural diuretics. If you have an issue with water retention, focus on adding more water-melon, dandelion greens, cucumber, parsley, and asparagus to your daily meals.

Group 4: Improving Cardiovascular and Metabolic Function

- **Heart:** Once you start to follow the detox diet, you may also notice that your blood pressure improves. That is because you are eating much less salt from processed foods and are eating much more veg-etables, which contain high amounts of potassium and magnesium, both well known to improve blood pressure. If you are concerned about high blood pressure, eat at least four stalks of organic celery each day. Also, make sure you are eating wild Alaskan salmon or sardines to get your omega-3 fatty acids, which help with choles-terol levels.

Group 5: Improving Hormone Balance

- **Endocrine:** If you have been previously diagnosed with hypothy-roidism, you will have one more reason to avoid soy in your diet. Also, you should be sure to eat cruciferous vegetables in modera-tion, because excessive consumption can worsen thyroid function.

Those same vegetables, however, are very effective at improving the detoxification of bad estrogens. The genus of vegetables known as brassica, or crucifers, includes broccoli, broccoli sprouts, kale, collard greens, cabbage, brussels sprouts, broccoli rabe, radish, arugula, watercress, and bok choy. The nutrients that help these foods to improve estrogen balance include a sulfur-containing compound called sulforaphane and another called diindolylmethane (DIM).

If you want to naturally improve thyroid function, eat more seaweed, which has iodine, one of the building blocks of the thyroid hormone. Also, you can use coconut oil in your salads, which has an impact on making the thyroid hormone more active.

The detox is just the beginning of lasting health. Now you will learn how to use this program as part of a greater lifestyle change or to reach weight-loss goals.

Conclusion

Day 31 and the Seven Steps to Lasting Health

After following the detox program and diet for thirty days, retake the detox questionnaire and check your weight. Compare your results to when you started the diet. In my study, patients reported that they generally lost about nine pounds and had a 66 percent reduction in symptoms after the initial thirty days. Hopefully, you will see just as much improvement.

This program can be the start of a whole new lifestyle. If you enjoyed the detox and are feeling significantly better but would still like to work on your weight, you can continue the program just as it stands until you achieve your weight-loss goal. You will continue to lose weight if you follow the diet as it was originally created, without the risk of losing important nutrients or starving yourself. You will also notice that the frequency and intensity of any remaining symptoms will continue to lessen the longer you stay on the program.

If you are not looking to lose more weight, I advise that you slowly begin to reintroduce the foods eliminated on the diet. This way, you will be able to clearly see which foods actually trigger an allergy or sensitivity. You can introduce one type of food at a time. For example, many of my patients are anxious to reintroduce the nightshade vegetables, including tomatoes and eggplants. Here's how to do it correctly: add tomatoes to one meal for one day. The following day, try to have tomatoes twice. If you don't experience any change in the way you look or feel, then you know that tomatoes do not cause an adverse reaction.

Continue with each of the nightshade vegetables until you have reintroduced all the ones that you enjoy. Then move to the next group of foods that you would like to try, and repeat the process. If you have a reaction to any type of food, do not continue to eat it. Make a note so that you remember which foods you are sensitive to, so you continue to avoid them in the future.

Meanwhile, try to continue to eat as many of the approved foods that you learned to enjoy on the plan, and stay away from the foods that caused you to have symptoms. It is not mandatory to reintroduce all the foods that you have eliminated. For example, if you find that you don't miss having coffee in the morning and now prefer green tea, then stick with your new routine. This is especially true with foods high in sugar. Hopefully, your sweet tooth will have diminished, so that you can stay away from toxic sugar as much as possible.

The ultimate goal of the detox diet is to restore your health and help you transition into a healthy lifestyle, so I encourage you to replace the shake with solid foods when you are ready. You can do this gradually: replacing one shake a day with a more balanced meal, even one from the meal plan. You can continue to use the shake for breakfast and have protein and vegetables for lunch, while maintaining similar snacks and dinner options. Many of my patients like the structure and ease of the shake, especially at breakfast. You can continue to have a daily shake indefinitely if you choose. The shake can also be an excellent choice for a midday snack.

Hopefully, you'll experience a change to a lifestyle that is more detox friendly. As part of your healthy lifestyle modification, you will want to continue to avoid processed, packaged, and canned foods and drinks, and other foods that are not freshly made. Continue to enjoy small fresh fish rather than larger, mercury-filled fish. Select organic produce, 100%

grass-fed meats, free-range chicken, and organic dairy products as often as possible. And while there are always a myriad of consumer products to choose from, select only those that will not reintroduce toxins back into your system or your home. Refer back to chapters 4 and 5 for reminders about which types of foods and products to buy and which to stay away from.

If after thirty days you do not experience any improvement in symptoms or loss of weight, this is a sign that you may have an underlying medical condition, like poor thyroid function. You should be checked by your doctor or health care provider to determine exactly what is going on with your health. Make sure to inform your doctor that you have been following this detoxification plan, so they know that you have already been attempting a diet modification to help improve your symptoms.

Recognizing Improved Health

By identifying the symptoms that toxins are causing, you took the first step toward better health. The next good decision was to follow the complete detoxification and learn how modifying your meal plan can help you feel better than you have felt in years. Now that you have completed your detox, you should hopefully be enjoying great results. You have allowed yourself the opportunity to heal, beginning at the cellular level. When your cells start healing themselves, you're literally going through an age-defying process, which not only improves your old symptoms but will increase your overall energy so that you no longer suffer from fatigue. You may notice that your brain fog has lifted and that you no longer have difficulty concentrating. Your hormone imbalances may also be corrected, and you'll start to look younger and feel younger as well. Your skin will be healthier. Your eyes will be brighter. People will start telling you that you look well or that you have taken five or ten years off of your age, and that's because you're healing yourself from the inside out.

At the same time, you might find that your mood has improved. You may be better able to deal with stressful situations because the food that you're eating is no longer adding another stress to your life. Just by improving your stress threshold, you are already supporting better health. And if you've lost weight, you may notice that you feel lighter, sleep better, and have more energy too.

I hope you have learned that aging does not equal illness or disease. You can grow old healthfully, and you can live a healthy life without necessarily needing to take prescription medications all the time. If you have embraced the detox, you now know that detoxing does not equal deprivation: you have been able to successfully rid your body of toxins without starving yourself or creating a stressful or uncomfortable situation. You have simply made small yet significant changes to the way you live. You now have all the tools you need to cleanse your body and clear your mind.

I also hope that you will share your experience with your friends and family, and with others who can benefit from hearing your story. Visit my Web site and let the entire detox community know how you've done over your 30-day program.

Seven Steps to Lasting Health

Each of these suggestions is meant to help improve mood and circulation while decreasing inflammation and toxic load. Together with the program, these seven steps are the building blocks to ongoing detoxification and represent a commitment to better health. While each has been described in detail several times, among other important tips and ideas, these are the backbone of any good detoxification program. If you can incorporate them into your daily life, you will find that the results of the detox will last longer. So even if you temporarily slip back into old habits, you will be able to maintain a much higher threshold before you begin to suffer from your body burden.

1. **Choose clean, organic, locally grown food:** Organic food has been shown to be higher in nutrients and lower in pesticides and insecticides than nonorganic foods. In addition, selecting locally grown food supports the livelihood of your community of independent farmers.

2. **Use water and air purifiers:** If you feel you are getting exposed to air- and waterborne pollutants, an air purifier and a water purifier can be very helpful for improving your health. They will lower your toxic exposures and thereby reduce your body burden.

3. **Exercise regularly:** Exercising regularly is a well-known way to improve your health. You will maintain and improve your muscle tone, maintain and improve your flexibility, and improve your mood. You will also improve circulation, which enhances detoxification; improve your ability to handle stress; and, of course, improve your metabolism.

4. **Get eight hours of sleep each night:** I can't overemphasize the importance of sleep for improving your health. During sleep your body has an opportunity to rest and heal itself from daily events. It is the prime time for liver detoxification, which is why it is ideal to have a bowel movement upon awakening or at least one bowel movement each day.

5. **Facilitate healthy digestive functions:** Your colon is your main route of toxin elimination. The longer it takes between bowel movements, the more likely you will reabsorb the same toxins that your liver is trying to eliminate. It is very important to have at least one to three bowel movements daily in order to optimize your detoxification process. The right diet, one that includes plenty of natural fiber, is the best way to aid the digestive process.

6. **Monthly dry saunas:** Our skin offers one of the most effective ways to eliminate heavy metals and fat-soluble toxins through sweating. When done correctly, saunas are a very safe and effective way to enhance the sweating process.

7. **Seasonal 10-day detox:** A seasonal 10-day detox gives you an opportunity to renew your health benefits on a regular basis. I recommend doing the short version of this same detox at the beginning of the spring, summer, and fall. Don't forget to take advantage of seasonal organic produce to make your detoxification more tasty and interesting.

The Bigger Picture

People just like you, all over the country, are beginning to recognize how detrimental chemicals and industrial pollutants are to our environment. The BP oil spill in the Gulf of Mexico in 2010 is just one example of how industries are inadvertently having a negative influence on the way we live and how they put our health and the health of our environment at risk.

The good news is that many companies are beginning to make significant changes in their manufacturing practices to try to decrease their environmental burden. Carpet companies, car companies, and paint companies, for example, are beginning to employ greener manufacturing processes, but we still have a long way to go. You can support the efforts responsible companies are making by using their environmentally friendly products: going green benefits us all.

The agriculture industry is still using a great deal of pesticides and insecticides and fertilizers that are not healthy for us or for the environment. Mercury is still being dumped into the water and winding up in the fish we eat. We're still getting exposed to the lead in old paint from before the 1970s and the lead that is still being used to manufacture bronze plumbing fixtures and is still found in water pipes. But now you have the knowledge about what these chemicals can do and how to avoid them.

I hope that this book will give you the ammunition and information you need to make wise and informed decisions, not only about what products to buy, but also about how to live a healthier life. It all starts with what we decide to put in our mouths. The meal plan is really the foundation for our health, and we have every opportunity to make the right decisions, which will, in turn, give our bodies a chance to heal themselves now and going forward.

Appendix I

Supporting Your Detox: Nutritional Supplements and More

In environmental medicine, the goal is to eliminate the cause of the problem, and then use a few specifically targeted, high-quality nutrient supplements to improve and optimize the body's capacity to work better and heal itself. Different supplements help the body accomplish and optimize the detox program and the subsequent healing process in different ways by providing it with all the nutrients it needs, in safe and effective doses. For each of the supplements listed, I will provide you with basic daily recommendations to get you started on the right track and give examples of manufacturers you may want to consider.

Because supplements are not as well regulated as conventional medicines, it is extremely important to purchase products that are high quality and free of fillers, flowing agents, artificial coloring, and artificial ingredients. In a congressional investigation reported by the *New York Times* in 2010, nearly all the supplements tested contained trace amounts of lead and other contaminants. Sixteen of the forty supplements tested contained pesticide residues that appeared to exceed legal limits.

Here's how to buy the best. Try to avoid products that include in their "other ingredients" any of the following: titanium dioxide, cornstarch, dextrin, polyethylene glycol (PEG), FD&C coloring, or dextrose. Look for products that are made to be hypoallergenic, "good manufacturing practice" (GMP) certified, and third-party tested for quality and consistency. You can find this information either by visiting the product manufacturer's Web site or by going to ConsumerLab.com (www .consumerlab.com), which has tested over two thousand supplements made by more than three hundred manufacturers.

Dr. Morrison's Preferred Supplement Manufacturers

There is no single company that has a perfect line of supplements. It's critical that you look at the back of the bottle, read through the "other ingredients," and make sure the product you are considering taking is clean. With that in mind, here are the companies I most often suggest to my patients.

Allergy Research Group	Metagenics
BioImmersion	Ortho Molecular Products
Bio-Tech Pharmacal	Perque
Daily Benefit	Researched Nutritionals
Douglas Laboratories	Thorne Research
Gaia Herbs	Vital Nutrients
Metabolic Maintenance	Xymogen

BEWARE OF TOXICITY IN HERBAL SUPPLEMENTS

Consumers truly need to be worried about the high levels of pesticides and heavy metals that can be found in some herbal products. The products most likely to be contaminated come from China and India. The best bet for consumers in the United States is to buy herbal supplements that are grown in the United States. Look for companies that manufacture products that do postproduction third-party testing on their products to ensure that they are free of contaminants.

Choose Supplements Based on Your Health Concerns

Depending on your initial response to the detox questionnaire, you may want to address specific health concerns with supplements during the 30-day program. Review your scores on the questionnaire and identify the body system with the highest relative score. Once you have found that section, take a look at the recommended supplements listed below for that body system and work with your health care provider to determine which supplements are right for you. Make sure to discuss whether these supplements will interfere with any medication you are currently taking. If you find that your symptoms have not improved or have worsened after you completed the 30-day detox diet and a supplement regimen, it is critical that you follow up with a health care provider to fully identify what is causing your symptoms. And please follow the safe, low doses that I recommend.

Group 1: Improving Neurological Function

The brain and nervous system can be very susceptible to the adverse effects of toxins. Based on the symptoms that you identified in the detox questionnaire, you may want to supplement with specific formulas that can improve your mood, lessen fatigue, and even decrease your anxiety or depression.

Decreasing Stress and Anxiety

When we are under acute stress, the body produces the adrenal hormone cortisol as well as the fight-or-flight hormone adrenaline (also known as epinephrine and norepinephrine). When stress becomes chronic and out of our control, the body can remain in an indefinite fight-or-flight response. The symptoms of this can include fatigue, anxiety, irritability, or even depression. The ideal scenario to manage chronic stress is to regain control of your life situation or find some type of outlet to relieve stress, such as exercise. However, while you are in the process of finding a long-term solution, supplements can be helpful in keeping your stress hormones balanced.

GABA (gamma-aminobutyric acid): An inhibitory brain chemical that helps balance energy-producing chemicals like epinephrine and norepinephrine. When you feel anxious, irritable, or overwhelmed, you may be experiencing an imbalance between the excitatory and inhibitory neurotransmitters. Some people deal with these symptoms by taking prescription medications like Valium, Ativan, or Xanax, which all work to calm the brain by interacting with GABA receptor sites. However, a more natural alternative is to directly take the amino acid GABA (500 mg daily) for symptom relief.

L-theanine: An extract of green tea and another GABA option that helps the body create more GABA on its own. I generally recommend 200 mg, in products such as Zen by Allergy Research Group, which contains 550 mg of GABA and 200 mg of L-theanine per two capsules (two capsules one to two times per day with food). Some people just take this at night to help with sleep.

Rhodiola rosea: A powerful adaptogen herb that is found in the polar region of eastern Siberia. The name "adaptogen" refers to the ability of an herb to adapt to your specific needs. For example, if a person requires a stimulating or calming action from the herb, it will work harmoniously with what your body needs. Rhodiola works as an adaptogen for the brain by promoting physical and mental energy. Choose a rhodiola product that is standardized to contain 3 percent Siberian *Rhodiola rosea* with bioactive rosavin, rosin, rosarin, and salidroside. I recommend Rosavin from Ameriden (two capsules in the morning with a meal).

Melatonin: When people are under chronic stress, sometimes the normal sleep-wake cycle gets disturbed. You may find that you have difficulty falling asleep or staying asleep. If you have tried the other recommendations I've made regarding better sleep but still need some additional assistance, the hormone supplement melatonin may be beneficial. Melatonin is made in the pineal gland, with peak levels occurring around 10:00 p.m. It can only be produced naturally when we sleep in a pitch-black room. If you sleep in a room that has enough light to allow you to see your hand when you wave it in front of your face with the lights off, then most likely you are not getting your required amount of melatonin and therefore you are not getting a deep night's sleep.

If you are also producing stimulating stress hormones or are in a pattern of staying awake late due to work or travel, taking a small dose of melatonin can be very helpful for getting to sleep successfully. Some people find that when they take melatonin they tend to get nightmares. I have found that the lower doses work better for sleep. I generally recommend melatonin spray (0.5 mg per spray, one spray under the tongue at bedtime).

Valerian and kava: Natural herbs that are very useful for helping to calm the brain and reduce stress. Valerian works like an herbal version of valium, without the side effects, and it is not addicting. The main drawback is that it smells like old socks. Kava also works well for anxiety and is less sedating than valerian. However, a few years ago kava got a bad rap, suggesting it caused liver toxicity. The problem with kava is not that it causes toxicity but that it can make other drugs you are taking more toxic. Do not take kava if you are on prescription medications. Look for valerian root standardized to 1.8 mg of valerenic acid and kava (or kava kava) standardized to 37.5 mg of kavalactones.

Licorice root (*Glycyrrhiza glabra*): An herb with many health benefits, including blocking cortisol breakdown. This is a good effect for someone with low blood pressure; however, licorice root can make high blood pressure worse, due to its ability to cause salt retention in the body. Look for a product that is standardized to 12 percent glycyrrhizin. I recommend the licorice root extract from Ortho Molecular Products (one capsule in the morning).

Reducing Fatigue and Improving Energy

Phospholipids and glycolipids: Special types of fats that are necessary for cell-membrane repair and proper cell-membrane fluidity. For our cells to produce energy properly, the mitochondria (the cells' power-houses) require intact membrane structure. By providing the correct phospholipids and glycolipids, the body is able to improve mitochondrial function, which in turn increases ATP production, which improves energy. In 2003 the *Journal of the American Nutraceutical Association* reported in a pilot study that a proprietary product called NT Factor was able to reduce fatigue by 33 percent in eight weeks. I recommend the product NT Factor from Researched Nutritionals (two capsules twice daily with food).

Vitamin B$_{12}$ (methylcobalamin): One of the most important vitamins for healing the nervous system. It is very effective for improving overall energy, mood, and memory. I always check blood levels of vitamin B$_{12}$ in patients who complain of poor concentration or brain fog, and I frequently find the levels to be low. Vitamin B$_{12}$ is naturally found in egg yolks and red meat. Vegetarians definitely need to go out of their way to ensure they do not become deficient, because there is no vegetable source for vitamin B$_{12}$. Also, as we get older we are not able to absorb vitamin B$_{12}$ as efficiently because it requires a low (acidic) stomach pH as part of the absorption process. I generally recommend liquid methyl B$_{12}$ (1,000 mcg under the tongue every morning for at least six weeks).

Improve Memory and Reverse Brain Fog

Phosphatidylcholine (PC): One of the most important components of the neuron cell wall, this supplement helps to maintain proper cell wall pliability and functions as one of the fats needed to maintain proper cellular communication. As we get older, this nutrient gets depleted and replaced in the nervous system with other less-flexible fats that cause cells to become stiff. The goal of taking extra PC is to help our neuronal cell walls heal themselves. While we can't grow new nerve cells, we can help the ones we have repair themselves.

Another important function of PC is to provide choline to make the brain chemical acetylcholine. Declining acetylcholine levels are thought to be the single most common cause for declining memory. This important fat is generally derived from egg yolks and from lecithin. You can also take 1,000 mg of PC from Thorne Research two times a day as a good way to provide the nutrition your brain needs.

Acetyl-L-Carnitine (ALC): L-carnitine's primary purpose is to shuttle fatty acids into the mitochondria (the cells' powerhouses) to be burned for energy. Many people take L-carnitine as a supplement to help with weight loss because it increases the amount of fat to be metabolized for energy. The addition of the acetyl group helps to make ALC fat soluble, so it can cross into the central nervous system more effectively, and the acetyl group can be used as a building block to make acetylcholine, the memory neurotransmitter, along with phosphatidylcholine. ALC is not found in any significant amount in food, but it can be taken as a supplement. I generally recommend taking 1,500 mg two times daily with food to improve memory, increase energy, and help with weight loss.

Group 2: Improving Immune Function

The part of the body with the most active immune function is the digestive tract, which not only digests and absorbs food but is also the first defense against bad bacteria, parasites, yeast, and other organisms that can enter our body during meals. In order to improve your whole body's immunity, the immunity in the digestive tract must be addressed first.

Probiotics: Good bacteria like acidophilus are one of the cornerstones of proper digestive function and proper digestive tract immune balance. Symptoms of imbalanced digestive bacteria include gas, bloating, constipation, and/or loose bowel movements. Some newly discovered probiotics, like VSL#3, may help with inflammatory bowel disease, while others have been found to eliminate the bacteria that cause traveler's diarrhea, like the good yeast *Saccharomyces boulardii*. Other probiotics, like *Bifidobacterium longum* and *Bifidobacterium lactis*, may improve metabolism.

Probiotics are naturally found in food that is fermented, such as yogurt, sauerkraut, and kimchi. These are also foods that are known to improve digestion and absorption of nutrients. Fermented beverages like beer and wine do not have good bacteria; instead they have yeast that turns sugar into alcohol.

The two probiotics that I recommend the most for improving digestive and immune function are Saccharomycin DF (two capsules in the morning) from Xymogen, and from Essential Formulas, Dr. Ohhira's Xtra Strength Professional Formula probiotic (two capsules at night).

Digestive enzymes: In addition to having the correct balance of good bacteria, it is also important to have an adequate amount of digestive enzymes in your stomach and small intestine to be available to properly digest protein, fats, and carbohydrates. Symptoms of low digestive-enzyme function can include reflux, heartburn, and abdominal bloating that occurs soon after a meal. Bloating that occurs after a protein-rich meal generally suggests low stomach acid. If the bloating occurs after a carbohydrate-rich meal, it generally suggests poor digestion of starches and fermentation of the starches lower in the digestive tract. Bloating after a fat-rich meal usually has to do with poor gallbladder function.

I recommend Metagest from Metagenics (one or two capsules before a protein-rich meal to improve digestion of meats and protein), Benezyme from Daily Benefit (one or two capsules after meals to aid in the digestion of vegetables and carbohydrates), and Digest RC (two capsules in the morning to improve gallbladder function and fat digestion). In addition, I often recommend a bitter herb product called berberine from Daily Benefit (one to two tablets two times per day) to help improve digestive function and to make the digestive tract inhospitable to bad bacteria and yeast.

Glutamine: The most important nutrient necessary to heal the intestinal lining and to improve immune system function. Glutamine generally is not considered an essential amino acid because we can synthesize it in our body when needed by breaking down muscle tissue. It happens to be the most abundant amino acid in the body, but at times of stress or illness the body can begin to break down muscle in order to meet the increased demand for glutamine to aid in repair. If our muscle mass becomes too depleted, then glutamine can become a conditionally essential amino acid: for example, when a person is severely ill and is not consuming enough animal protein, they may require glutamine supplementation.

Additionally, the immune system is highly dependent on glutamine for proper functioning. You should be suspicious that you are glutamine deficient if you have any type of chronic digestive symptoms or any type of chronic disease or illnesses. Also, if you are a vegetarian, you should consider supplementing the glutamine in your diet.

I generally recommend using Glutamine Plus from Daily Benefit (two teaspoons in three ounces of water at least once daily). This supplies about 7,000 mg of glutamine per serving. It also has two anti-inflammatory herbs to help heal the digestive tract: deglycerized licorice and nonbitter aloe.

IgG 2000: A highly purified, dairy-free immunoglobulin supplement from Xymogen. By taking one tablespoon twice daily you can support your immune function, reduce inflammation in the digestive tract, begin to heal gut permeability, and neutralize major pathogens.

Cordyceps sinensis: A unique fungus that has been used for centuries in traditional Chinese medicine. This fungus is an adaptogen that can be immune stimulating, meaning it can boost your immune system; and immune balancing, meaning that it can be used for autoimmune disease. It is known to protect liver and kidney function and to boost blood production. Look for a cordyceps extract that is standardized to an adenosine level of at least 0.2 percent. I generally recommend Cordimmune because it's produced in a lab and is free of heavy metals and chemicals (take two capsules in the morning).

Plant sterols and sterolins: Sterols are plant fats that have immune-balancing effects. Sterolins are plant compounds that make the sterols work better. A great deal of research has been conducted on how these plant compounds act like adaptogens to balance immune system function. The research has suggested the correct ratio of sterols to sterolins to achieve the optimal results in autoimmune and inflammatory conditions is one hundred to one. The supplement I recommend, which has the plant sterols in the suggested ratios, is Moducare (two capsules in the morning and one capsule at night, on an empty stomach).

Detoxing the Lymphatic System

The lymphatic system is the circulatory system for your immune system. It is responsible for moving lymph (the combination of immune cells and toxic waste) out of body tissue and back to general circulation for processing. Inflammation decreases the efficiency of this process and can even stop it. Reducing inflammation is one of the best ways to improve the function of the lymphatic system and help your body remove toxins properly.

Proteolytic enzymes: These help to reduce inflammation in the tissue by neutralizing and breaking down the chemicals that cause it. The enzymes must be taken on an empty stomach at least thirty minutes before meals or two hours after meals. I recommend Vascuzyme from Ortho Molecular (three tablets two times a day, before meals).

Turmeric and curcumin: Spices that have long been used for their anti-inflammatory effect. Turmeric contains curcumin, both of which work as antioxidants and anti-inflammatory agents. Turmeric and curcumin have both been used in cooking, but in this form they are not well absorbed into the body. A curcumin extract that does absorb well and that I recommend is Meriva-SR from Thorne Research (two capsules daily). This is a supplement and should not be used for cooking.

Lungs

To keep the lungs functioning optimally it is important to control both inflammation and bronchospasm (spasm in the bronchial muscles).

Glutathione: An antioxidant that is produced in every cell of the body to combat inflammation and to improve cellular detoxification. Glutathione is synthesized from the amino acids L-cysteine, L-glutamine, and L-glycine. During periods of extreme stress or under a heavy body burden of toxins, the body may not be able to produce enough to meet every cell's needs. Taking glutathione as a supplement would seem like an obvious solution; however, glutathione is not very well absorbed when taken orally because it gets broken down into its precursor amino acids in the digestive tract. Recently, a new delivery system has been developed involving the use of the beneficial fat phosphatidylcholine, which helps glutathione be absorbed orally. There is a growing body of evidence that suggests that glutathione can help decrease the inflammation in lung conditions. The product I recommend is called liposomal glutathione (one teaspoon twice daily or more often, depending on your needs).

N-acetylcysteine (NAC): This has received a good deal of press lately because it has been found to help fight off the H1N1 flu. Research has shown that NAC helps reduce hospitalization among people suffering from chronic obstructive pulmonary disease, according to a study in the *European Respiratory Journal*. It also helps to prevent chronic bronchitis, or inflammation in the lungs. When taken in higher doses, it works like a natural decongestant and mucolytic, which helps move mucus out of the lungs. One of the reasons NAC works for inflammation in the lungs is that it helps your body to make glutathione. I recommend taking the 600 mg NAC from Metabolic Maintenance (two capsules two times a day).

Quercetin: A plant-derived bioflavonoid and the natural pigment found in grapefruit, onions, apples, and black tea. It mainly functions as an antioxidant and at a high dose can prevent the release of histamine from mast cells. This means that it is helpful for allergies and decreasing inflammation, especially in the lungs and upper airway. I recommend using 500 mg quercetin (two capsules two to three times per day, with food, for at least three weeks).

Buffered vitamin C: This works like an antioxidant to help decrease inflammation. "Buffered" refers to the fact that minerals like calcium, magnesium, and potassium are added, to make it less acidic. Research has shown that people with asthma may require less inhaled medication if they take vitamin C, according to the journal *Respiratory Medicine*. Studies have also shown that taking vitamin C before an athletic event can decrease the risk of exercise-induced asthma. By taking buffered vitamin C, you also get the minerals that can help prevent broncho-spasm from occurring. Because of the serious nature of asthma, please work with your health care provider before you modify your lung medications. I recommend using the 720 mg buffered vitamin C capsules from Daily Benefit (take two daily with food) or Potent C Guard powder by Perque (take one-half teaspoon in three ounces of water).

Skin

Vitamin A: Deficiency in vitamin A can cause skin rashes. If you have a chronic inflammatory skin condition, including acne, vitamin A may be a helpful supplement for your symptoms. Vitamin A is fat soluble, so it can build up to toxic levels and caution must be taken when dosing. If you smoke cigarettes, take vitamin C with vitamin A to minimize your chance of lung cancer. Also, pregnant women should not take more than 10,000 IU of vitamin A daily (otherwise there is an increased risk of birth defects).

I recommend taking buffered vitamin C (720 mg daily) with 25,000 IU of micellized vitamin A (daily for at least six weeks). Do not take higher doses or a longer continuous course, unless you are working with a health care provider.

Methylsulfonylmethane (MSM): A sulfur-containing nonessential amino acid that is touted for its anti-inflammatory activity. It is also an important building block for skin and connective tissue, and is used extensively by the liver to improve sulfur-dependent detoxification processes. MSM is very safe to use, even at high doses. I recommend taking 2,000 mg of MSM (one tablet three times per day with meals).

Silica: One of the most abundant minerals in the earth's crust, it is also extremely important for proper connective-tissue and collagen synthesis. Orthosilicic acid (H_4SiO_4) is easily absorbed and seems to have the best results for skin, hair, nail, and tissue healing. You may need this if you find that you have dry or fragile skin, or soft or brittle nails, or bruise easily; all of which are symptoms of toxicity or the inability to absorb certain nutrients. To get the most active form of silica, I recommend RegeneMax from Xymogen (two 5 mg capsules daily).

Group 3: Improving Weight Loss and Digestion

One of the most important processes during detoxification is to have at least one to three bowel movements daily. The colon is the exhaust system of your body, so if you are not moving your bowels regularly, it doesn't matter how well your liver processes the toxins you encounter. If the colon is backed up, your liver will back up, which in turn puts more stress and pressure on other routes of detoxification like the kidneys or skin.

Magnesium oxide: A poorly absorbed version of magnesium that can help to improve bowel movements without acting like an aggressive stimulant. It is safe to use over long periods of time, without adverse effects. It can be easily dosed by following these simple guidelines. If you take magnesium oxide at night and you do not have a complete evacuation the next morning, you did not take enough. If the next morning the bowel movement is loose, you took too much. I generally recommend beginning with a very easily dosed version, 3A Magnesia (take three to six 200 mg tablets at bedtime).

Improve Liver Function

Milk thistle (silymarin): Milk thistle has been used as an herbal remedy for thousands of years. It is thought that the active ingredient is a flavonoid called silymarin. It helps protect the liver because of its antioxidant, anti-inflammatory, and reparative properties. However, milk thistle can cause certain prescription medications to become more toxic, including antipsychotics, Dilantin, allergy drugs, statins, antianxiety drugs, blood thinners, and some cancer drugs. If you are taking any of these drugs, you should not take milk thistle. When I use this product, I recommend Silymarin Forte (80 percent silymarin) from Ortho Molecular (two 200 mg capsules at night).

Glutathione: One of the most important antioxidants for the body, it is probably the most important antioxidant for the liver. When the body is under stress from toxic exposures, the demand for glutathione rises. It plays an important role in phase-two liver detoxification, especially in helping the body deal with toxic heavy metals. If our cells do not produce adequate amounts of glutathione to meet our needs, then our body becomes toxic. By taking an absorbable version of glutathione orally, you can meet your daily needs. I recommend liposomal glutathione (one teaspoon twice daily mixed in three ounces of water).

Improve Kidney Function

Optimal kidney function can only occur if you also have a well-functioning digestive tract and colon. The supplement I believe works the best to improve kidney function is asparagus, which is known to help alkalinize the body for better detoxification, and it helps to improve the digestion and absorption of nutrients from the stomach and intestinal tract. I recommend Chi's Enterprise asparagus extract, which is extracted from whole, organically grown asparagus (mix one bag with warm water two times per day before meals).

Group 4: Improving Cardiovascular and Metabolic Function

The two most important methods of detoxing your cardiovascular function are to control inflammation and improve vasodilation (opening of the blood vessels). Below are some nutrients that you may want to consider.

Omega-3 fatty acids: Polyunsaturated fatty acids (PUFAs) are essential to proper human function. We must get these fats from our diet because the body cannot create them on its own. Omega-3 fatty acids include alpha linolenic acid (ALA), eicosapentaenoic acid (EPA), and docosahexaenoic acid (DHA). Omega-3 fatty acids are important in our diet because as our food has become more processed the level of omega-3 fatty acids has fallen considerably. Also, we have become accustomed to eating grain-fed cows and chickens that are no longer producing meat with high levels of this essential PUFA. Omega-3s are anti-inflammatory and protect against heart disease.

ALA is found in both plant (flaxseed, chia seed, walnuts) and animal sources (oily fish like salmon and halibut as well as 100% grass-fed beef and free-range chicken eggs). As we age, our body has a more difficult time converting the ALA found in foods into the active EPA and DHA. For this reason, many people benefit from taking fish oil supplements to get the active form.

In addition, an important omega-6 fatty acid has become depleted as well. Gamma-linolenic acid (GLA), which is found in borage and evening primrose oils, works synergistically with the omega-3s to optimize the anti-inflammatory effect. If you want to have the most complete anti-inflammatory omega-3, it should be combined with GLA. I recommend taking Nordic Naturals Pro EFA Extra (one capsule twice daily with meals). Another option is Barlean's cold-pressed flaxseed oil (one tablespoon together with a 300 mg GLA capsule twice daily with food).

Lumbrokinase: A fibrinolytic (able to dissolve fibrin blood clots) enzyme that is produced from earthworm extract. It does not affect the blood-clotting cascade, so it can be used safely with blood-thinning medications. It works for people who are prone to blood clots or are hypercoagulable due to some underlying infection, illness, or toxicity that causes inflammation that affects the proper flow of blood through capillaries. It has been used safely in Chinese medicine for thousands of years and has been well researched in the Chinese literature. For circulatory health, I recommend taking Boluoke (one 200 mg capsule twice daily on an empty stomach: thirty minutes before meals or two hours after meals).

Magnesium: One of the most important minerals for proper body function. It is necessary for over 250 different enzymatic processes in the body, such as normal energy function, muscle function, and helping to normalize blood pressure. Yet at times of stress, magnesium is quickly used and depleted from our body. In order to get an easily absorbed form of magnesium, it should be bound to a protein molecule. I recommend Mag Glycinate from Daily Benefit (two 100 mg capsules at bedtime).

Improving Heart Function

Coenzyme Q_{10} (CoQ_{10}): A substance that is naturally produced in the body and a mandatory component in the production of cellular energy. It is found in mitochondria: the cells or organs with the highest energy demands—like the heart, brain, and liver—have the highest CoQ_{10} concentrations. When our cells become toxic, they have more difficulty producing CoQ_{10} and as a consequence the cells function at a lower level of capacity. Symptoms of poor CoQ_{10} production (a.k.a. mitochondrial dysfunction) include fatigue, poor stamina, and difficulty concentrating. Also, patients with congestive heart failure can benefit from taking CoQ_{10}.

I recommend a water-soluble version of CoQ_{10} called Chew Q (100 mg) from Daily Benefit (one tablet daily). Another very good option is the preconverted active form of CoQ_{10}, ubiquinol (take 100 mg daily). For severe mitochondrial dysfunction, I recommend Researched Nutritionals CoQ_{10} (up to three 400 mg capsules daily).

B vitamins pyridoxine (B_6), methylcobalamin (B_{12}), and folic acid: Necessary for the conversion of the cardiovascular toxic amino acid homocysteine to its nontoxic precursor methionine. If homocysteine levels build up to an abnormally high level for a period of time, you can be susceptible to forming blood clots. By taking vitamin B_6 (100 mg), vitamin B_{12} (1,000 mcg), and folic acid (1 mg) all together, you can lower your homocysteine levels. I recommend taking Cardio B from Ortho

Molecular (one capsule daily) and checking your homocysteine levels every three months until you get a reading of less than 10.

D-ribose: Studies suggest that D-ribose can restore energy and improve function in ischemic, hypoxic, and failing hearts. In addition to improving cardiac function, D-ribose can increase energy levels for people with chronic fatigue syndrome and fibromyalgia. I recommend RibosEnergy from Researched Nutritionals (one scoop added to four ounces of liquid twice daily).

Improving Endocrine Function

There are some very good supplements that may be able to assist in keeping blood sugar balanced and improve insulin sensitivity. For example, cinnamon has been shown to reduce fasting blood-sugar levels after forty weeks of using as little as one-quarter teaspoon daily, which is why I include it in the detox shake. Cinnamon is also found in a concentrated form called Cinnulin PF (a twenty-to-one extract of cinnamon).

Chromium picolinate: A trace mineral that is important in transporting sugar from the bloodstream into cells to be used as energy. It is mostly found in whole grains, spices (black pepper, thyme), and mushrooms, and it is depleted from foods during the refining process. To replenish the trace mineral in your diet, it is recommended to take chromium picolinate (500 mcg) daily.

Banaba leaf extract: Considered to have the potential to improve blood-sugar control through an active ingredient called corosolic acid.

To improve blood-sugar levels, I recommend a product that has all three of these ingredients, Cinnulin PF, chromium picolinate and banaba leaf extract, GlucoBenefit from Daily Benefit (one capsule twice daily with food).

Alpha-lipoic acid (ALA): A unique antioxidant that is both water soluble and fat soluble. This trait allows this molecule to easily cross through cell membranes and through the blood-brain barrier. It is effective in regenerating vitamins C and E, it increases glutathione levels, and it helps to prevent DNA damage. Research has recently identified its mechanism of action for improving insulin sensitivity. An article in *Diabetes Technology & Therapeutics* showed that taking 600 mg of ALA daily for twelve weeks reduced C-peptide levels, an indication of increased insulin sensitivity. I recommend taking ALAmax CR from Xymogen (one tablet twice daily with food). If you are taking blood-sugar lowering medicines, please only use this under the supervision of a health care provider who can safely monitor your blood-sugar levels.

Group 5: Improving Hormone Balance

Diindolylmethane (DIM): A naturally occurring phytonutrient that is found in cruciferous vegetables like broccoli, brussels sprouts, and cabbage. It is believed to help improve estrogen balance by improving the liver's ability to metabolize unhealthy estrogen levels. This enables DIM to decrease the incidence of hormone-related symptoms, like premenstrual syndrome, fibrocystic breast disease, fibroids, and even prostate enlargement. I recommend taking DIM (75 mg) twice daily with food.

Borage oil: Borage is a plant with blue star-shaped flowers. The oil extracted from the seeds contains high amounts of the omega-6 fatty acid GLA (gamma-linolenic acid), which has anti-inflammatory properties by working with omega-3 fatty acids to create a hormone-like substance called prostaglandin E_1 (PGE_1). GLA is known for improving inflammatory conditions, including PMS. I recommend taking GLA (300 mg) twice daily and fish oil (1,000 mg twice daily with food). If you are a vegetarian, substitute cold-pressed flaxseed oil (one tablespoon twice daily) for the fish oil.

Sulforaphane: A naturally occurring compound, found in high concentrations in broccoli seeds, that possesses antioxidant activity and improves phase-two liver detoxification. Scientists at Johns Hopkins discovered this extract in 1992 and found that there was a correlation between sulforaphane intake and a lower incidence of cancer. It is thought that this works by helping the body to properly metabolize estrogen, thereby improving proper hormone balance. I recommend Oncoplex from Xymogen (one capsule twice daily with food).

While they aren't supplements per se, the following additional treatment options can, in conjunction with the detox program, help improve specific symptoms.

Consider Chelation Therapy

If you believe that heavy metals may be contributing to your high blood pressure, heart disease, or problems with chronic inflammation, talk with your doctor to see if you are a candidate for chelation therapy. This treatment option works like an antioxidant for removing heavy metals from the body: it blocks free-radical-producing electrons from causing damage, and it also becomes a vehicle to move the metal out of the tissue, into the bloodstream, and out of the body. Chelation therapy has been used for treating heavy metal accumulation, including iron toxicity, and to treat acute toxicity from lead.

This type of therapy is not for everyone and is only administered by a licensed health care provider. It involves the administration of a semi-synthetic amino acid either orally or intravenously on a regular interval over weeks or months. The oral chelating agent generally used is called DMSA or Chemet; the intravenous chelating agent is called EDTA or versenate. For more information, or to find a doctor that specializes in chelation, visit the American College for Advancement in Medicine Web site (www.acam.org).

Consider Counseling

Often during the course of an effective detoxification emotional issues come up and need to be addressed. These issues can be just as devastating to your health as physical toxins. They can stem from an adverse experience from childhood or the recent past. These experiences have an impact on how the body can heal itself. I have seen time and again that when a patient reaches a plateau during their detoxification process, it may be because the emotional component of their health has not been adequately addressed.

The following are specific types of counseling that I often recommend to my patients and that you might be interested in exploring:

Somatic Experiencing: A guided therapy performed by trained psychiatrists, therapists, and social workers and aimed at resolving the physical manifestations of emotional stress or trauma. This therapy is useful for posttraumatic stress disorder (PTSD), breaking the cycle of repetitive unhealthy behaviors, and chronic pain conditions.

Eye movement desensitization and reprocessing (EMDR): A comprehensive form of psychotherapy performed by psychiatrists, therapists, and social workers that is useful for relieving symptoms resulting from disturbing and unresolved life experiences. This is useful for people suffering from PTSD.

Emotional Freedom Technique (EFT): A form of psychotherapy that attempts to manipulate the body's energy fields by tapping on acupuncture points while focusing on a specific traumatic memory, with the goal of alleviating the problem.

Spiritual healers: They attempt to balance the emotional, spiritual, and physical energy within a person to restore total body balance. Specially trained rabbis, priests, and doctors perform this work.

Appendix II

Questions for Your Doctor and Additional Testing Options

We all know that the typical doctor's office visit is less than ten minutes. So in order to make the most of your time, you need to be prepared with a list of questions to ask your doctor. The purpose of these questions is to see if your physician is open to exploring environmental exposure as a potential cause of your current symptoms and/or conditions.

Question 1: Are you open to this detoxification strategy? Whether you are responding well to your current treatment or if you feel that you should be doing even better, you may want to discuss your plans to follow this program with your doctor. This will help the doctor to monitor your progress and have the best picture of your current health.

Question 2: If my score on the detox questionnaire was low, what types of preventative laboratory tests should we be running? Standard preventative tests include the CBC (complete blood count) and CMP (comprehensive metabolic panel) as well as tests for certain nutritional deficiencies like 25-OH vitamin D, vitamin B_{12}, folic acid, ferritin (iron storage), and RBC-Mg (magnesium is important because it's the most commonly depleted mineral in the body due to stress and poor food choices). If heart disease runs in your family or you are concerned about heart disease, you may want to take the advanced lipid panel (through Berkeley Heart Lab) or VAP and also screen for additional risk factors like homocysteine, lipoprotein (a), and hs-CRP (high-sensitivity C-reactive protein). Additionally, I would recommend checking blood Hg (mercury) and Pb (lead) levels as a screening test.

Question 3: If my symptoms are not getting better, would you be open to doing these additional tests? For the most part, doctors will have either one of two reactions. The first is, "Okay, let's just do the test. I don't have enough time to even think about it. Let's just see what comes back and if there's a problem, then we'll take it from there and refer you to somebody who can take care of it."

Or they might say, "Look, your insurance is not going to cover it. It's not conventional testing, and I'm just not going to do it for you." If this happens, you will have to try to find another resource for this testing. Two valuable Web sites list doctors across the country that may be open to doing these types of tests: the American College for the Advancement in Medicine (www.acam.org) and the American Academy of Environmental Medicine (www.aaemonline.com).

Symptom-Specific Tests

You can confirm your results from the detox questionnaire with a variety of laboratory tests that your doctor can order. These tests include blood work, saliva, urine, skin, and stool testing. The following tests are grouped into general categories that will help you and your doctor to look for an underlying cause of your symptoms. Many of these tests are part of a traditional health workup, and can be done through routine labs.

However, some tests may need to be ordered by an integrative-medicine physician through specialty labs and may be considered as part of a nonconventional or complementary approach. Your doctor might not be familiar with some of these tests. However, it's recommended that you work with your physician to see if they're open to exploring this type of testing, and if they aren't, you may want to consider finding another doctor who is more receptive to this approach to run these specialized tests.

Work with your health care provider to individualize your testing based on your circumstances and current health. These suggestions should not take the place of a thorough medical evaluation. Other tests may need to be ordered that are not part of the list.

Group 1: Neurological Testing

- **Urine test:** NeuroScience Neuro-focus Test (measures epinephrine, norepinephrine, serotonin, and dopamine). The company Neuro-Science (www.neurorelief.com) has developed a test to determine your balance of neurotransmitters. You can work with your health care provider to access these tests.

- **Blood tests:** vitamin B_{12}, folic acid, 25-OH vitamin D, whole blood mercury (Hg), whole blood lead (Pb), red blood cell magnesium (RBC-Mg), Genova DetoxiGenomic Profile

Group 2: Immune Testing

Allergy Testing

- **Blood tests:** serum IgE; ImmunoCAP for food, environmental, and mold allergies; Metametrix IgG4 food-allergy test; antigliadin antibody; antiendomysial antibody; antitransglutaminase antibody (for gluten sensitivity); MELISA test (for allergy to metals)

- **Skin tests:** provocation/neutralization testing (P/N testing) to specific antigens or allergy triggers (e.g., foods, molds, pollen)

Inflammation Testing

- **Blood tests:** erythrocyte sedimentation rate (ESR), high-sensitivity C-reactive protein (hs-CRP), antinuclear antibody (ANA)

Infection Testing

- **Blood tests:** complete blood count (CBC)
  - If tick bite suspected: IGeneX or SUNY Stony Brook Lyme Western Blot IgG, IgM; babesia antibody IgG, IgM; bartonella antibody IgG, IgM; ehrlichia antibody IgG, IgM
  - If chronic infections: Epstein-Barr virus (EBV) titer, human herpesvirus 6 (HHV-6) titer, cytomegalovirus (CMV) titer

Group 3: The Digestive Workup

- **Stool tests:** Genova Comprehensive Digestive Stool Analysis and Parasitology (CDSA/P) test (for assessing digestion and absorption of food and parasite presence), Hemoccult (for assessing blood in stool), Metametrix GI Effects stool analysis (for assessing digestion and absorption of food and parasite presence)

Group 4: Cardiovascular and Diabetes Testing

The Cardiac Workup

- **Blood tests:** advanced lipid panel (through Berkeley Heart Lab) or VAP, homocystine, high-sensitivity C-reactive protein (hs-CRP), fibrinogen, lipoprotein (a), ferritin, whole blood, mercury (Hg), whole blood lead (Pb)

The Diabetes Workup

- **Urine test:** complete urinalysis (UA)
- **Blood tests:** fasting blood sugar, hemoglobin A₁C, GlycoMark, five-hour glucose tolerance test with insulin levels (GTT) (a five-hour GTT is the best way of looking not only for diabetes but also for insulin resistance and hypoglycemia)

Group 5: Gender-Specific Health Concerns

Blood Tests

- **The female workup:** estradiol, total estrogen, progesterone, testosterone, DHEA-S
- **The male workup:** estradiol, testosterone, DHEA-S, PSA
- **The stress workup:** 9:00 a.m. cortisol, pregnenolone, DHEA-S
- **The metabolic workup:** TSH, Free T3, Free T4, antithyroid antibodies, 9:00 a.m. cortisol

Saliva Tests

- **The stress workup:** adrenal health test (measures cortisol and DHEA levels)

Specific Testing for Toxic Sensitivities

- **Testing for toxic chemical exposure:**
  - Blood tests: Metametrix PCBs Profile, Metametrix Chlorinated Pesticides Profile, Metametrix Volatile Solvents Profile

- Urine Tests: Metametrix Porphyrins Profile, Metametrix Phthalates & Parabens Profile

● **Testing for heavy metal exposure:**
  - Blood tests (for recent exposure): blood mercury (Hg), lead (Pb), cadmium (Cd), arsenic (As), aluminum (Al)
  - Urine tests (for accumulation or storage): Doctor's Data twenty-four-hour urine toxic elements (on the same day draw the blood work for heavy metals and collect urine after taking a binding agent such as DMSA; this helps clarify if current or old exposure)

Appendix III
Additional Resources

- For more information about recognizing and managing pesticide poisoning, visit the pesticides homepage on the EPA's Web site (http://www.epa.gov/pesticides/index.htm).
- For help identifying all types of pollutants, visit the Environmental Working Group (EWG) Web site (www.ewg.org).
- A great resource for natural pest control options can be found at Eartheasy (http://eartheasy.com/non-toxic-pest-control).
- EWG's cosmetics database helps you choose safer personal care products. In addition to generating a hazard score (on a one to ten scale), it allows you to search by brand and for products without certain ingredients or health effects.
- A great deal of information on the health consequences of plasticizers and endocrine disruptors can be found at TEDX (www.endocrinedisruption.com), a site founded by one of the nation's top research scientists on this matter, Dr. Theo Colborn.
- An excellent resource to purchase 100 percent grass-fed beef is at U.S. Wellness Meats (www.grasslandbeef.com).
- For coconut salad-dressing ingredients, such as coconut aminos (a vinegar substitute), try Coconut Secret (http://www.coconutsecret.com/aminos2.html).

References

Chapter 3

Gatto, N., M. Cockburn, J. Bronstein, A. D. Manthripagada, and B. Ritz. "Well-Water Consumption and Parkinson's Disease in Rural California." *Environmental Health Perspectives* 117 (2009): 1912–18.

EPA, "List of Air Toxics in the 2002 NATA Assessment" accessed at http://www.epa.gov/ttn/atw/nata2002/02pdfs/2002polls.pdf.

Chapter 5

Gao, Y., and E. Charter. "Nutritionally Important Fatty Acids in Hen Egg Yolks from Different Sources," *Poultry Science* 79, 6 (2000): 921–24.

Chapter 7

Gaby, A. "The Role of Hidden Food Allergy/Intolerance in Chronic Disease." *Alternative Medicine Review* 3, 2 (1998): 90–100.

Ascherio, A., H. Chen, M. G. Weisskopf, et al. "Pesticide Exposure and Risk for Parkinson's Disease." *Annals of Neurology* 60 (2006): 197–203.

Trasande, L., P. Landrigan, C. Schechter, et al. "Public Health and Economic Consequences of Methylmercury Toxicity to the Developing Brain." *Environmental Health Perspectives* 113 (2005): 590–96.

Jusko, T., C. Henderson, B. Lanphear, et al. "Blood Lead Concentrations <10 mcg/dL and Child Intelligence at 6 Years of Age." *Environmental Health Perspectives* 116 (2008): 243–48.

Chapter 8

Bagenstose, L., P. Salgame, M. Monestier. "Murine Mercury-Induced Autoimmunity in Mice: A Model of Chemically Related Autoimmunity in Humans." *Immunologic Research* 20, 1 (1999): 67–78.

Chapter 9

Phillips, M. "Gut Reaction: Environmental Effects on the Human Microbiota." *Environmental Health Perspectives* 117, 5 (2009): 198A–205A.

Guarner, F., and J. Malagelada. "Gut Flora in Health and Disease." *Lancet* 361, 9356 (2003): 512–19.

Baillie-Hamiton, P. "Chemical Toxins: A Hypothesis to Explain the Global Obesity Epidemic." *Journal of Alternative and Complementary Medicine* 8, 2 (2002): 185-192.

Chapter 10

Depalma, R. G., V. W. Hayes, B. K. Chow, et al. "Ferritin Levels, Inflammatory Biomarkers, and Mortality in Peripheral Arterial Disease: A Substudy of the Iron (FE) and Atherosclerosis Study (FeAST) Trial." *Journal of Vascular Surgery* 51, 6 (2010): 1498–1503.

Bao, B., A. S. Prasad, F. W. Beck, et al. "Zinc Decreases C–Reactive Protein, Lipid Peroxidation, and Inflammatory Cytokines in Elderly Subjects: A Potential Implication of Zinc as an Atheroprotective Agent." *American Journal of Clinical Nutrition* 91, 6 (2010): 1631–41.

Lin, J., D. Lin-Tan, K. Hsu, and C. Yu. "Environmental Lead Exposure and Progression of Chronic Renal Diseases in Patients Without Diabetes." *New England Journal of Medicine* 348 (2003): 277–86.

Chapter 11

Williams, G. "The Role of Oestrogen in the Pathogenesis of Obesity, Type 2

Diabetes, Breast Cancer, and Prostate Disease." *European Journal of Cancer Prevention* 19, 4 (2010): 256–71.

Chapter 12

Gardner, C., A. Kiazand, S. Alhassan, et al. "Comparison of the Atkins, Zone, Ornish, and LEARN Diets for Change in Weight and Related Risk Factors among Overweight Premenopausal Women." *Journal of the American Medical Association* 297 (2007): 969–77.

Index

Acetylcholine, 240
Acetylcholinesterase (AChE), 56
Acetyl-L-carnitine (ALC), 241
N-acetylcysteine (NAC), 188, 245
Acidophilus, 153, 155, 241
Acne, 5, 41
Acupuncture, 20, 138
Adaptation, 18–19
Adipocytes, 149
Adrenaline, 92, 93, 121, 172, 182, 200, 237
Aerobic exercise, 171
AGE (advanced glycation end product), 105–106, 196
Agricultural waste, 34
Air contamination, 48–53
Air fresheners, 60, 62, 63
Air pollution, indoor, 59–61
Air purifiers, 60–61, 231
Alcohol, 199
Algae, 42, 53
Allergies, xiii, 41, 122–124, 126, 176
    affect on overall health, 130–132
    distinguished from cold, 6–7
    food (see Food allergies)

hygiene hypothesis and, 123, 129
infant feeding and, 130
mercury and, 71–73
testing, 257–258
Alpha hydroxyl acids, 64
Alpha linolenic acid (ALA), 249
Alpha-lipoic acid (ALA), 106, 251–252
Alternative and Complementary Therapies, xv
Alternative Medicine Review, 47
Aluminum cans, 45
Aluminum cookware, 196
Aluminum foil, 197
Alveoli, 7
Alzheimer's disease, 106, 196
American Academy of Environmental Medicine, xvi, 256
American College for the Advancement of Medicine, 256
American College of Sports Medicine, 38
American Dental Association, 71, 134–135
American Heart Association, 44
American Medical Association, 64

Amino acids, 98, 187–188, 202
Ammonia, 64
Anabolic hormones, 175
Anaerobic metabolism, 103–104
Anaphylaxis, 83
Andropause, 112, 174, 175
Anemia, 53, 167
Ankylosing spondylitis, 123
Annals of Neurology, 114
Antacids, 152, 153
Antibacterial products, 61, 64, 79, 123
Antibiotics, 37, 85, 118, 120, 126, 133, 152
Antidepressants and anti-anxiety
    medications, 117
Antihistamines, 126
Antimicrobials, 145
Antinuclear antibodies (ANA), 134
Antioxidants, 18, 46, 47, 106–108, 145,
    158, 188, 220, 224, 244–245, 252
Anxiety, xi, 112
    supplements and, 237–239
Apple cider vinegar, 155
Arachidonic acid, 97
Aromatization, 177
Arsenic, 34, 68, 97
Arthritis, xi, 127
Artificial sweeteners, 221
Asbestos, 51, 59
Aspergillus, 75
Associated Press, 34
Asthma, 7, 19, 20, 49–51, 122, 126, 246
Atherosclerosis, 102, 146
Athletes
    anaerobic metabolism, 103
    meal plan for, 211–212
Athlete's foot, 77
Ativan, 238
Atkins, Robert, xvi, 206
Atkins diet, 189
Atopic eczema, 130

A TO Z Weight Loss Study, 204
ATP (adenosine triphosphate), 103–104,
    109, 161, 240
Attention deficit disorder (ADD), 112,
    131, 176
Attention deficit hyperactivity disorder
    (ADHD), 131, 176
Autism, increase in, 176
Autoimmune disease, 21, 84, 122–123,
    126, 134
Autonomic nervous system, 114, 182

Babesia, 118, 133
Bacteria, 37, 46, 81, 122, 123, 142–143,
    150–153
Bacteroidetes, 143
Bactrim, 57
Baillie-Hamilton, Paula, 148
Baking soda
    bathing in, 140–141
    as household cleaner, 62, 63
Banaba leaf extract, 251
Bartonella, 118, 133
Basic Olive Oil Vinaigrette, 219–220
Bathing, 139–141
Batteries, 69
Beans, 96, 207–208
Beef, grass-fed, 41, 46, 97, 169
Beets, 207, 223
Belching, 150
Benfotiamine, 106
Benzene, 38, 51, 52–53
Berberine, 242
Beta-carotene, 207
Betaine, 207
BHA, 64, 145
BHT, 145
Bifidobacillus, 153
Bile, 10, 157
Binge eating, 142

Biochemical individuality, 20–21
Biological pesticides, 57
Bioplastics, 42, 73
Birth defects, 38, 51, 246
Birth weight, 40
Bisphenol A (BPA), 21, 41–42, 45, 73, 74, 148–149, 173
Bitter herbs, 156
Bladder, 9
    inflammation, 127
Bloating, xiii, 10, 30, 81, 84, 146, 150
Blood-brain barrier, 114, 116
Blood-sugar levels, 10, 92–93, 120–121, 163–165
Blumberg, Bruce, 149
Body burden, 3–16
    genetics and, 4, 15–16
    kidneys, 8–9
    liver, 9–10
    lungs, 7–8
    lymphatic system, 11
    nose and upper airway, 6–7
    skin, 5–6
    stress, 13–14
    symptoms of toxicity and, 21–22
    weight gain, 11–13
Body mass index (BMI), 54, 165, 211, 212
Boluoke, 249
Borage oil, 252
Borax, 62, 63
Borrelia, 133
Bottles
    plastic baby, 41, 148
    water, 35, 73, 74
Bowel movements, 151, 152, 200
    number of, 10, 156, 231, 247
    unhealthy, 10
Bragg Sea Kelp Delight Seasoning, 219
Brain, xii, 12, 111–121

infections affecting, 118–120
    inflammation in, 116–117
    toxins poisoning, 113–116
Brain fog, 112, 113, 119, 120, 240–241
Braly, James, 86
Braverman, Eric, 223
BRCA1/BRCA2 genes, 15
Breads, 93–94
Breast cancer, 15, 34, 42, 64, 95, 174
Breast milk, 130, 174, 176
Breathing, 3, 137–138
Brominated fire retardants (BFRs), 66
Bromine, 37
Bronchi, 7, 8
Bronchial asthma, 130
Bronchial tree, 7
Bronchitis, 49–51
Bronchoconstriction, 38
Building material outgassing, 59

Cadmium, 51, 52, 68, 72, 123, 134, 135, 136
Caffeine, 45, 96, 220, 221
Calcium, 109, 166, 188
Calories, 13, 192, 193, 204
Cancer, xii, 15, 19, 34, 38, 40, 41, 51, 82, 110, 195, 252–253. (see also specific cancers)
Candida, 118
Carbamate pesticides, 56
Carbaryl, 56
Carbofuran, 56
Carbohydrates, 15, 102, 142, 163–164, 192, 201, 202
Carbon, 35, 36, 38
Carbon air purifiers, 60
Carbon dioxide, 7, 105, 137
Carbon filters, 38
Carbon monoxide (CO), 48, 49
Cardiac workup, 258–259

Cardiovascular and metabolic function
  on detox questionnaire, 27
  supplements and, 248–252
Cardiovascular disease, 160–162. (*see also* Heart disease)
Cardiovascular testing, 258–259
Carpet, removing old, 66
Carrots, 207
Castile soap, 62, 63
Cast-iron cookware, 63, 79, 196–197
Catalase, 108
Cataracts, 106
Celery, 207, 223
Celiac disease, 86, 87
Cells, 101–110
  AGE (advanced glycation end
    product) and, 105–106
  free radicals and, 108
  function of, 102
  oxidative stress and, 107–108, 166
  oxygen and, 103–104
  water and, 108–109
Cellular dysfunction, 18, 36, 104–106
  detoxification and, 109–110
Cellulite, 11
Cellulose, 76
Centers for Disease Control and
    Prevention (CDC), 115, 176
Central nervous system, 38, 113, 115, 119
Ceramic cookware, 197
Chelation therapy, 253
Chemotherapy, 116, 178, 179
Chest pain, 8, 161
Chlordane, 56, 150
Chloride, 109
Chlorine, 37–38, 123, 142, 143, 150
Chlorpyrifos, 56
Cholesterol, 165, 166, 168, 170–171, 225
Chromium picolinate, 251
Chromosomes, 173

Chronic fatigue syndrome, xi, 21, 104,
    107, 110, 251
Chronic rhinitis, 130
Cigarette smoking, 19, 52, 59, 168, 246
Cinnamon, 202, 203, 251
Circulation journal, 168
Cladosporium, 75
Clean Air Act, 49
Cling wraps, 74
Cocaine, 142
Coenzyme Q10 (CoQ10), 250
Coffee, 96, 107, 194, 220–221
Colds
  distinguished from allergies, 6–7
  symptoms, 84
Cold water plunge, hot water followed
    by, 172
Coliforms, 36
Colitis, 127
Colonic hydrotherapy, 157–158
Colonoscopy, 87
Community supported agriculture
    (CSA), 48
Complex carbohydrates, 163
Concentration, xiii, 12, 21, 84, 107, 113
Constipation, 10, 36, 151, 152
Construction sites, 50
Cooking, 196
Cookware, 63, 79, 196–197
Copper, 188
Cordyceps sinensis, 243
Corn, 96
Coronary artery disease, 161
Corosolic acid, 251
Cortisol, 30, 181–182, 237
Costume jewelry, cadmium in, 72
Coughing, 7, 8, 19, 124
Counseling, 253–254
Crinnion, Walter, 47
Crohn's disease, 122

Curcumin, 244
Cyrus, Miley, 72
L-cysteine, 245
Cystitis, 127

Dairy products, 19, 41, 224
  elimination diet and, 90–91, 94–95,
    126, 133
  food sensitivities and, 85, 155
  hormones added to, 45
  mucus production and, 6
  organic, 48
Dangerous Grains (Braly), 86
DDT, 56, 149, 150
Dehydration, 146, 151, 166, 221
Dementia, 112, 116
Dental fillings, mercury in, 70–72, 116,
    118, 134–135, 143
Dental fluorosis, 57–58
Dental health, 15–16
Deodorants, 64
Depression, xi, 93, 112
Detergents, 53
Detox diet (*see* Detoxification program)
Detoxification program, xi, xiii, 124,
    127, 130–133, 144, 146, 147, 153,
    154, 178–179
  benefits of, xiv, 190–191
  clinical paper on, 188–190
  costs of, xv
  detox protein shake, 186, 187–188,
    189, 202–206, 212, 228
  eating out, 198–199
  getting ready for, 185–200
  meal plan (*see* Meal plan)
  questionnaire, 22–29, 89, 124, 132,
    147, 155, 170, 179, 181, 189,
    191–192, 201, 227
  sleep and, 199–200
  supplements (*see* Supplements)

10-day plan, 29–30, 195, 232
30-day plan, 29, 107, 119–120,
    192–193
  withdrawal process and, 92, 191
Developmental disorders, 41
DHEA, 182
Diabetes, xi, xiv, xv, 9, 15, 92, 106, 110,
    160, 163–165, 165
Diabetes Technology & Therapeutics, 252
Diabetes workup, 259
Diamino benzene, 64
Diaphragm breathing, 137–138
Diarrhea, 10, 36, 150, 151
Dieldrin, 150
Diet and nutrition, xiv, xvii, 4, 33. (*see
    also* Meal plan)
  carbohydrates, 15, 102, 142, 163–164,
    192, 201, 202
  cravings, 120, 152, 201, 202
  dairy products (*see* Dairy products)
  dental health and, 15–16
  eating out, 198–199
  fiber, 10, 51, 155–156, 231
  fish (*see* Fish)
  fruits and vegetables (*see* Fruits and
    vegetables)
  gluten, 85–89
  grass-fed beef, 41, 46, 97, 169
  organic food, 41, 45–48, 55, 193, 201,
    228–229, 231
  processed foods, 91, 92, 106, 142, 144,
    145–147, 163–165, 224
  protein, 96–97, 102, 163, 192, 208,
    212, 213
  raw foods, xv, 152, 153
  seasonal foods, 31, 195–196, 208, 232
Diethyltoluamide (DEET), 57
Digestion, 3, 4, 9, 81–82, 85, 120, 126,
    127, 142, 143, 150–159, 224,
    241–243

Digestive enzymes, 154, 242
Digestive workup, 258
Diindolylmethane (DIM), 226, 252
Dimercaptosuccinic acid (DMSA), 72
Dioxins, 15, 40–41, 150, 173
Dish soaps, 62
Disinfectants, 37, 53, 61, 150
DL-methionine, 202
DNA (deoxyribonucleic acid), 15, 105
Docosahexaenoic acid (DHA), 97, 249
Dopamine, 111, 114, 142, 223
Drain cleaners, 62
D-ribose, 251
Dry brushing, 137
Dry cleaning, 51
Dry sauna therapy, 5

Ear infections, 86
Eating out, 198–199
Eat Well Guide, 208
Eczema, 5, 126, 130
Eggs, 45, 97, 131
Ehrlichiosis, 118, 133
Eicosapentaenoic acid (EPA), 97, 249
Electrical pollution, 67–68
Electromagnetic Biology and Medicine, 67
Electronics, PBDEs in, 66–67
Electron transport chain, 105
Elimination, xiv, 3, 4, 200. (*see also*
    Bowel movements)
Elimination diet, 89–90, 131. (*see also*
    Detoxification program)
  dairy products, 90–91, 94–95, 126
  gluten, 86–88
  goal of, 90
  grains and breads, 93–94
  meal plan (*see* Meal plan)
  nightshade vegetables, 95–96
  reintroducing foods, 227–228
  sugar, 91–93

Emotional freedom technique (EFT), 254
Emphysema, 49–51
Endocrine disruptors, 41–42, 64,
    173–175, 220
Endocrine system, 173, 251–252
Endometriosis, xv
Endorphins, 172
Environmental Health Perspectives, 53,
    115, 143
Environmental medicine, xvi, 19, 32.
    (*see* Detoxification program)
Environmental Protection Agency
    (EPA), xii, 33, 38–40, 48, 49, 51
  Web sites of, 36, 49, 70
Environmental toxins, 32–58
  air contamination, 48–53
  food supply, 39–47
  in home (*see* Home, eliminating
    toxins in)
  pesticides (*see* Pesticides)
  symptoms of toxicity (*see* Toxicity,
    symptoms of)
  water contamination, 34–42
Environmental Working Group (EWG),
    54, 65, 79
Epigenetics, 15
Epinephrine, 111, 237, 238
Epsom salts, bathing in, 139
Esophageal sphincter, 151
Estrogen, 147, 173–175, 177
*European Journal of Applied
    Physiology*, 104
*European Journal of Cancer
    Prevention*, 180
*European Journal of Clinical
    Nutrition*, 94
European Respiratory Journal, 245
Exercise, 231
  aerobic, 171
  cellular dysfunction and, 104

Exercise-induced asthma, 38, 246
Exfoliation, 140
Eye movement desensitization and
reprocessing (EMDR), 254

Familial health patterns, 15
Farm runoff, 36, 53
Fasting blood sugar, 165, 170
Fat, dietary, 102, 145, 163
Fat cells, 12, 53–54, 115, 149
Fatigue, xiii, 41, 112, 113, 119, 150
    supplements and, 239–240
Fatty liver, 164, 178
Fatty tumors (lipomas), 11
Ferritin levels, 167, 170, 255
Fertility, 38
Fertilizers, 34, 47, 52, 232
Fetal development, 173–174, 176
Fiber, 10, 51, 155–156, 231
Fibroblasts, 149
Fibromyalgia, xi, 21, 104, 107, 110, 195
Fight-or-flight hormone, 93
Fire retardants, 66–67, 79
Firmicutes, 143
Fish, 33, 40, 97, 102, 225, 228
    benefits vs. risks, 44
    cleaning and cooking, 150
    mercury in, 42–44, 102, 116, 118,
        169, 232
Fish oil supplements, 44, 193, 249
Flaxseed, 156, 202, 203, 252
Fluid retention, 12, 13, 30, 84, 109, 143,
    145, 146, 225
Fluoride, 57–58, 150
Fluoropolymer, 196
Folic acid, 250, 255
Food, Inc. (movie), 46
Food allergies, xvi, 4, 82–83, 130, 144.
    (see also Elimination diet)
    differed from food sensitivities, 83–85

fruit, 95
milk, 94–95
symptoms of, 83
Food and Drug Administration (FDA), 47
    Web site, 43, 116
Food sensitivities, xvi, 4, 82–83. (see also
    Elimination diet)
    differed from food allergies, 83–85
    symptoms of, 84
Food supply
    environmental toxins and, 39–47
    genetically modified organisms
        (GMOs), 46–47
    hormones added to, 45, 177
    pesticides in, 53–55
    preservatives in, 46, 80, 91
Formaldehyde, 62, 64
Formula, infant, 130
Free radicals, 108, 167
Fruit pectin, 156
Fruits and vegetables, 201, 206–210,
    213, 222–226
    allergies to, 95
    local and organic (see Organic food)
    nightshade vegetables, 95–96, 133,
        134, 213, 227–228
    pesticides in, 55, 102
Fungicides, 53
Furans, 40–41
Furniture and floor polish, 62, 63

GABA (gamma-aminobutyric acid),
    111, 223, 238
Gallbladder, 10
Gallstones, 202
Garlic, 156
Gasoline, 38, 49, 167
Gastritis, 154
Gastroplasty (bariatric surgery), 54
Genetically engineered hormones, 45

Genetically modified organisms
(GMOs), 46–47
Genetics, 4, 15–16, 17, 122
GLA (gamma-linolenic acid), 249
Glassware containers, 197
Glucagon, 92, 121
Glucose, 9, 103, 105, 163
Glutamine, 242–243
L-glutamine, 202, 245
Glutathione, 71, 244–245, 248, 251
L-glutathione, 188
Glutathione peroxidase, 108
Gluten, 85–89
Gluteomorphin, 86
L-glycine, 202, 245
Glycogen, 163, 164
Glycolic acid, 64
Glycolipids, 239–240
Grains, 207–208
Green tea, 45, 188, 193, 221
Ground-level ozone, 49, 50
Growth hormone, 45

Hair dyes, 64, 70
Hair growth, excessive, 177
Hardening of arteries, 102, 146
Harvard School of Public Health, 114
Hashimoto's thyroiditis, 82, 84
Hazardous air pollutants (HAPs), 51–53
Heart arrhythmia, 162
Heart attack, 162, 168
Heartburn, 151, 156
Heart disease, xiv, xv, 9, 15, 21, 50, 106, 110
    death rate from, 162
    inflammation and, 161–162, 166–167
    lead levels and, 168
    linked to diabetes, 165
    preventative laboratory tests and,
        255–256
    symptoms of, 161–162

Heating and cooling systems, 59
Heavy metals, xii, xv, xvi, 5, 21, 36,
    50, 109, 112, 123. (see also Lead;
    Mercury)
    chelation therapy and, 253
    detoxification and, 135–136
    exposure in home, 68–73
    inflammation and, 134–135
    mineral imbalance and, 166–167
    in supplements, 235, 236
    testing for exposure to, 260
Hemochromatosis, 167
Hemorrhoids, 10
Heptachlor, 56
Herbicides, 34, 53
Herbs, 156, 159, 223
High blood pressure, xi, xiv, xv, 9, 15,
    21, 50, 69, 102, 162, 165, 168
    improving, 225
    reversing, 169–171
High-efficiency particulate air (HEPA)
    purifiers, 60, 78–79
Hispanic descent, 15
Hives, 5
Home, eliminating toxins in, 59–79
    cadmium, 72
    electrical pollution, 67–68
    fire retardants, 66–67
    heavy metals, 68
    household cleaners, 62–63
    indoor air pollutants, 59–61
    lead, 68–69
    mercury, 69–73
    mold, 75–79
    personal care products, 64–65
    plastics, 73–74
    reading product labels, 65
Homeopathy, 20
Homeostasis, 102, 109
Homocysteine, 250, 256

Homogenization process, 94, 95
Hormone imbalance, xi, xii, 21, 112, 147, 173–182
   chemotherapy and, 178, 179
   on detox questionnaire, 27–28
   improving, 225–226
   infertility, 176
   insecticides and pesticides, 175
   meditation and, 182
   sugar and, 177–178
   supplements and, 252–253
   testosterone and, 180–182
Hormone replacement therapy, 147, 148, 178
Hot tubs, 172
Household cleaners, 33, 60, 62–63
Houseplants, 75
hs-CRP, 167
Human body (*see* Body burden)
Hybridization, 85, 86
Hydrochloric acid, 153, 154
Hygiene hypothesis, 123, 129
Hypertension (*see* High blood pressure)
Hyperventilation, 8
Hypoglycemia, 92
Hypothyroidism, 225
Hysterectomy, 179

IgE-related allergy, 83
IGF-1 (insulin-like growth factor), 95
IgG 2000, 243
Immune function
   on detox questionnaire, 24–26
   improving, 122–141, 224
   supplements and, 241–247
   symptoms of failed, 128–129
Immune response, 82–84, 114, 116–117
Immune system, 7–8, 41, 81, 224
Immune testing, 257–258

Indigenous cultures, dental health and, 15–16
Indigestion, 151, 152
Indoor air pollutants, 59–61
Industrial waste, 15, 35, 102
Infections, 4, 5, 107, 122, 126, 156
   inflammation and, 133–134
Infection testing, 258
Infertility, xii, 174, 176, 177
Inflammation, 5, 7, 90, 95, 131–132
   diseases related to, 125
   heart disease and, 161–162, 166–167
   heavy metals, 134–135
   as immune response, 123–124
   infections, 133–134
   of joints and muscles, 134
   parasites and, 152
   sugar and, 143–144
   supplements to decrease, 136
   switch phenomenon and, 126–127
   symptoms of, 128–129
Inflammation testing, 258
Inorganic chemicals, 36
Inorganic mercury, 70
Insecticides, 52, 53, 56–57, 109, 112, 173, 232
Insect repellents, 57
Insoluble fiber, 156
Insomnia, 113
Institute for Responsible Technology, 47
Insulin, 120, 163–164
Insulin levels, 92
Insulin resistance, 91, 164, 177
Interstitial fluid, 109
Intestinal gas, xiii, 10, 81, 151
Ionic air purifiers, 60, 61
Iron, 47
   cellular oxidation and, 166
   levels of, 167
Irritability, xi, xiii, 21, 93, 112, 113, 146

Irritable bowel syndrome, xi, 107, 152
Itchy eyes and ears, 7
Ivermectin, 57

Jacuzzis, 172
Joint problems, 50, 86, 95, 119, 126, 127, 132–133, 135, 136
Journal of Alternative and Complementary Medicine, 148
Journal of the American Medical Association, 168, 204
Journal of the American Nutraceutical Association, 240
Journal of Vascular Surgery, 167
Juicing, 222–223

Kava, 239
Kenner, Robert, 46
Kidneys, 5, 30, 225
    damage, 9, 38, 52, 106
    drainage remedies, 159
    function of, 8–9, 13, 248
Kwell, 56

Laboratory tests, preventative, 255–257
Lactic acid, 64, 103–104
Lactose intolerance, 94
Lancet, 131
Lead, 21, 34, 135, 136, 232, 256
    brain and, 114–116
    cellular oxidation and, 107, 166
    exposure in home, 68–69, 169
    levels of, 167–168
    sources of poisoning, 49–50
    steps to reduce exposure, 169
    symptoms of poisoning, 69
Leaky gut syndrome, 81–82, 95
Learning disabilities, 40
Lecithin, 202–203, 241
Lemon juice, 62, 63

Lice, treatment for, 56–57
Licorice root (*Glycyrrhiza glabra*), 239
Lindane, 56
Liver, 5, 30, 164–165, 188, 224
    damage, 38, 41, 52
    function of, 9–10, 13, 247–248
Loofah sponge, 140
Lumbrokinase, 249
Lung cancer, 36, 246
Lungs, 7–8, 137–138, 224, 244–246
Lyme disease, 78, 118, 119, 133, 135
Lymphatic drainage, 137
Lymphatic system, 11, 109, 131, 137, 244
Lymph edema, 109
L-lysine, 202

Mad Hatter syndrome, 115
Magnesium, 47, 68, 71, 109, 139, 166, 188, 250, 255
Magnesium oxide, 247
Malathion, 56
Male menopause, 112
Martial arts, 182
Meal plan, 186, 201–226
    acceptable foods, 208–210
    for athletes, 211–212
    beverages, 220–222
    foods to avoid, 213–214
    juicing, 222–223
    personalizing, 223–226
    salad dressings, 218–220
    sample 30-day, 214–217
    sea vegetables, 210
    for vegetarians, 212
Meat, 206–207
    grass-fed beef, 41, 46, 97, 169, 207
    hormones added to, 45, 177
Meditation, 182
Medium-chain triglycerides (MCTs), 188, 223

Melatonin, 200, 238–239
Memory changes, xi, xiii, 12, 40, 50, 86, 107, 117–118, 240–241
Menopause, 112, 135, 168, 174, 179
Menstrual cycles, 21, 40, 174, 176, 177
Mercury, xi, 21, 51, 69–73, 97, 123, 256
  allergic reactions and, 71–73
  autoimmune disease and, 134–135
  brain and, 114–116
  as cause of cellular toxicity, 70–71
  cellular oxidation and, 107, 166
  in dental fillings, 70–72, 116, 118, 134–135, 143
  detoxification, 117–118
  disposing of products containing, 70
  elemental, 69–70
  in fish, 42–44, 102, 116, 118, 169, 232
  symptoms of poisoning, 42–43
Metabolic syndrome, 161, 165, 170, 172
Metabolism, xii, 11, 46, 148, 175, 212, 241
Metallothionein, 71, 115
Metametrix PCBs Profile, 41
Methylene chloride, 51
Methylmercury (organic mercury), 42, 70
Methylsulfonylmethane (MSM), 246
Microbial pathogens, 36
Microwave cooking, 198
  in plastic containers, 33, 41, 74, 79
Migraine headaches, 130
Mildew, 62, 63
Milk, 94–95, 131
Milk thistle (silymarin), 247–248
Mirex, 56, 150
Mitochondria, 103–105, 108, 109, 161, 240, 250
Molds, xvi, 19, 46, 53, 59, 62, 63, 79, 118
  allergic reactions to, 76
  brain and, 119

  common, 75
  evaluating home for, 76–78
  symptoms of toxicity, 119
  toxic, 76
Molecular mimicry, 122–123
Mononucleosis, 83
Mood swings, 112, 113, 120, 146
Morphine, 142
Motor vehicle exhaust, 40, 49, 51, 52
Mountain Valley Spring Water, 35
Mouth/throat, on detox questionnaire, 25
MTBE (methyl tert-butyl ether), 38–39
Mucosal epithelium, 6
Mucus, 6–8, 85
Mud and clay packs, 140
Multiple sclerosis, 194
Multivitamins, 193
Murphy Oil Soap, 63
Muscle aches, xiii, 50, 103–104, 119
Muscle cramps, 166
Mycotoxins, 76

Nail polish and removers, 64
Nasal infections, 84–85
National Health and Nutrition Examination Survey, 168
National Listing of Fish Advisories database, 39
Native Americans, 15
Natural cleaning options, 62–63, 79
Nausea, 151
Nephropathy, 165
Nerve damage, 106
Neurodegeneration, 116
Neurological development, 41
Neurological function
  on detox questionnaire, 23–24
  improving, 223
  supplements and, 237–241
Neurological symptoms, 111–121

Neurological testing, 257
Neuropathy, 165
Neurotoxicity, 116
Neurotransmitters, 111, 117
Newbold, Retha, 148
New York Times, 34
Nickel, 71, 135, 197
Nicotine, 107
Nightshade vegetables, 95–96, 133, 134, 213, 227–228
9/11 terrorist bombings, 50
Nitrates, 38, 50
Nitrogen dioxide, 50
Nonstick cookware, 63, 196, 197
Norepinephrine, 111, 237, 238
Nose, 6–7, 84–85
NT Factor, 240
Nutrition (*see* Diet and nutrition)
Nutritional supplements (*see* Supplements)

Oat bran, 156
Obesity, xi, xiii, 41, 160–161. (*see also* Weight issues)
    pesticides and, 54, 148, 149
Oily skin, 5
Omega-3 fatty acids, 44, 97, 145, 169, 193, 223, 224, 225, 248–249
Omega-6 fatty acids, 145, 249, 252
Opioids, 142
Oranges, 131
Organ damage, 36
Organelles, 103
Organic bedding, 66
Organic chemicals, 35–40
Organic food, 13, 41, 45–48, 55, 193, 201, 228–229, 231
Organic Foods Production Act, 47
Organic Trade Association, 48
Organochlorine, 54

Organochlorine insecticides, 56–57
Organophosphates, 56
Osteoarthritis, 134
Osteoporosis, 194, 197
Ovarian cancer, 42, 64, 178
Over-the-counter medications, 9
Oxidative stress, effects of, 107–108
Oxygen, 7, 49, 103–105, 161
Oxygenates, 38
Ozone air purifiers, 60
Ozone pollution, 49, 50
Ozone treatments, 38

Packaging, 45
Paint, lead-based, 50, 68, 69
Pancreas, 163, 164
Parabens, 64, 173
Parasites, 36, 37, 123, 150, 151–154
Parasympathetic nervous system, 31, 182
Parkinson's disease, 53, 114
Particulate matter, 50
Passing gas, 150
Pasteurization, 94
Penicillium, 75, 118
Perchloroethylene, 51
Perfluoroalkyl compounds, 149
Peripheral nervous system, 113, 114
Permethrin, 57
Peroxide, 64
Personal care products, 60, 64–65, 79
Pesticides, 9, 34–36, 47, 102, 109, 112, 123, 150, 173, 232
    in antibacterial products, 61, 64
    brain and, 114
    fat cells and, 53–54
    health concerns and, 54
    increase in use of, 54
    list of foods containing, 54–55
    obesity and, 54, 148, 149

Parkinson's disease and, 53
sexual health and, 175
types of, 56–58
Pharyngitis, 123
Phosphatidylcholine, 202, 240–241
Phospholipids, 239–240
Phosphorus, 47
Phthalates (plasticizers), 15, 41, 45, 64,
   73, 149, 173
Placenta, 173
Plankton, 40, 42
Plants, 75, 79
Plastic containers, 33, 41, 74, 79, 197
Plasticizers, 15, 41–42
Plastics, safest, 73–74, 79
Plastic shopping bags, 41
Plastic wrap, 42, 197
Pollution, xi, 33
   air, 49–53
   electrical, 67–68
   water, 34–35, 39–40
Polybrominated diphenyl ethers
   (PBDEs), 66
Polychlorinated biphenyls (PCBs), 40,
   149, 150
Polycystic ovary syndrome (PCOS), 177
Polystyrene, 73
Polytetrafluoroethylene (PTFE), 196
Polyunsaturated fatty acids (PUFAs),
   248–249
Polyurethane foam products, 66
Polyvinyl chloride (PVC) plastics, 73
Post nasal drip, 6
Posttraumatic stress disorder (PTSD),
   254
Potassium, 109, 166, 204, 221
Pottery, 69
Poultry, hormones added to, 45, 97
P-phenylenediamine, 64
Preconception detoxification, 176

Prednisone, 30
Premenstrual syndrome, 252
Prescription binding agents, 72
Prescription medications, xv, 9, 20, 124,
   126, 153, 154, 172, 238, 247
Preservatives, xii, 46, 80, 91, 145
Price, Weston, 15–16
Probiotics, 154, 155, 194, 241–242
Processed foods, 91, 92, 106, 142, 144,
   145–147, 163–165, 224
Product labels, reading, 64–65
Progesterone, 147, 173, 174
Prostaglandin E1 (PGE1), 252
Prostate cancer, 34, 42, 64, 174, 180
Protein, 96–97, 102, 163, 192, 208, 212,
   213
Protein powder, 187, 202
Proteolytic enzymes, 244
Psoriasis, 5
Psyllium husk, 156, 202, 203
Puberty, early onset of, 42, 64
Pur Advantage pitcher, 37
Pyrethrin, 57
Pyrethroid pesticides, 57
Pyrex cookware, 63, 79

Quercetin, 106, 245

Radiation, 36
Radioactive elements, 34, 36
Radishes, 156
Radon, 36
Raw foods, xv, 152, 153
rBGH (recombinant bovine growth
   hormone), 45, 95
Red blood cells, 8, 9, 53
Reflux, 151, 153–155
Refreshing Mint and Olive Dressing,
   219
Reproductive disorders, 38, 40, 51

Respiratory Medicine journal, 246
Restaurants, 198–199
Retinopathy, 165
Retroperitoneum, 8
Rheumatoid arthritis, 82, 84, 122, 123, 134
Rhodiola rosea, 238
Ringworm, 77

Safe Drinking Water Act, 34
Salad bars, 152
Salad dressings, 218–220
Saliva tests, 259
Salt, 91, 146, 151
Saltwater pools, 38
San Francisco Bay Regional Water Quality Control Board, 39
Saponins, 95, 96, 134
Saratoga Spring Water Company, 35
Saunas, 5, 72, 138–140, 231
Sea salt, bathing in, 139
Seasonal affective disorder, 194–195
Seasonal foods, 31, 195–196, 208, 232
Sea vegetables, 210
Secondhand smoke, 19
Seeds, 96
Selenium, 68, 71, 188
Septic tanks, 36
Serotonin, 111, 120
Sewage, 34, 36, 37
Sex hormones, 173–175, 179
Shopping bags, plastic, 41
Shortness of breath, 8, 162
Silica, 246–247
Simple carbohydrates, 163
Sinus congestion, 6, 126
Sinuses, 6, 19, 86
Sinus infections, 126
Skin, 5–6, 138–140
Skin care products, 15

Skin rashes, 5, 41, 52, 86, 126, 135, 224, 246
Sleep, 199–200, 231, 238–239
Slim-Fast, 189
Smog, 49
Smoking, 19, 52, 59, 168, 246
Sneezing, 7
Soda bottles, 45
Sodium, 109, 166, 204, 221
Sodium nitrite, 145
Soluble fiber, 156
Somatic experiencing, 254
Sore throat, 123, 144
Soy products, 96, 131, 212, 225
Spices, 133, 223, 244
Spicy Flax Dressing, 220
Spiritual healers, 254
Spreading phenomenon, 19
Spring cleansing, 30–31
Sprouted-grain breads, 93–94
Stachybotrys, 76, 118
Stainless steel cookware, 63, 79, 197
Steroids, 120, 126, 152
Sterols and sterolins, 243–244
Stevia, 221
Stomach problems, 36, 151
Street drugs, 9, 142
Strep throat, 123, 124
Stress, 4, 5, 13–14, 180–182, 200, 230
  supplements and, 237–239
  symptoms of chronic, 14
Stroke, 106, 162, 168
Stuffy nose, 6
Styrene, 38
Styrofoam, 42, 73
Sugar, 107, 131
  addiction to, 92, 142
  AGE (advanced glycation end product) and, 105–106
  avoidance of, 91–93

craving for, 120, 152
food sensitivities and, 85
in fruits, 208
hormone imbalance and, 177–178
inflammation and, 143–144
Sugarcane, 92
Sulfates, 50
Sulfites, 145
Sulforaphane, 226, 252–253
Sulfur dioxide, 51
Sullivan, John, xv
Sunscreen, 195
Superfund, 39
Super-oxide dismutase, 108
Supplements, 4, 28, 72, 124, 166, 186,
    193–195, 235–253. (see also specific
    vitamins)
    cardiovascular and metabolic
        function and, 248–252
    fish oil, 44, 193, 249
    hormone imbalance and, 252–253
    immune function and, 241–247
    neurological function and, 237–241
    preferred manufacturers, 236
    products to avoid, 235
    weight loss and digestion and,
        247–248
Sushi, 152
Svetol, 194
Sweating, 3, 5, 138, 231
Sweet Basil and Flaxseed Oil Dressing, 218
Swelling, 12, 123, 137, 143, 144
Swimming pools, chlorine alternatives
    for, 38
Switch phenomenon, 20, 126–127, 130
Sympathetic nervous system, 114
Systemic lupus, 82, 122, 134

Tai chi, 182
Taurine, 188

Teas, 221–222
Teflon-coated nonstick pans, 63, 196, 197
Temperature of body, 5
Testosterone, 174–175, 177, 180–182
L-theanine, 238
Thimerosal, 70
3-3 Dressing, 219
L-threonine, 202
Throat infections, 84–85, 123
Thyroid function, 225–226, 229
Thyroid hormone, 182
Tick bites, 118, 133, 134
Tin cans, 45
Toenail fungus, 77
Toilet bowl cleaners, 62
Toluene, 51
Toxicity, symptoms of, 17–31
    adaptation, 18–19
    biochemical individuality, 20–21
    body burden and, 21–22
    spreading phenomenon, 19
    switch phenomenon, 20
Toxic mold stachybotrys, 76
Trachea, 7
Traditional Chinese medicine, 138, 243,
    249
Transaturated fats, 102
Tributyltin, 149
Trichloroethylene (TCE), 38, 51–52
Triclosan, 64
Triglycerides, 44, 165, 170
Trihalomethanes (THMs), 35–37
Tub and tile scouring powder, 63
Turbinates, 6
Turmeric, 244

Ubiquinol, 250
Ultraviolet techniques, 38, 61
Université Laval, 54
Upper airway, 6–7

Uranium, 34, 36
Urinary tract infections, 124, 143
Urination, 200
Urine, color and smell of, 9

Valerian, 239
Valium, 238
Vegetables (*see* Fruits and vegetables)
Vegetarians, 240, 243, 252
  meal plan for, 212
Ventilation, poor, 59, 60
Vitamin A, 188, 246
Vitamin B, 9, 188
Vitamin B$_1$, 106
Vitamin B$_6$ (pyridoxine), 250
Vitamin B$_{12}$ (methylcobalamin), 240,
  250, 255
Vitamin C, 47, 169, 194, 246
  buffered, 245–246
  flush, 158
Vitamin D, 8, 188, 194–195
Vitamin D$_3$, 169
Vitamin E, 188
Volatile organic compounds (VOCs),
  35, 38–39, 50, 51
Vomiting, 151

Waste incineration, 40
Water bottles, plastic, 35, 73, 74
Water contamination, 34–42
Water intake, 108–109, 199, 220
Water purifiers, 37, 231

Wax paper, 197
Weak spot, 123–124, 135
Weight/digestion function, on detox
  questionnaire, 26–27
Weight issues, 11–13, 84, 107, 142,
  147, 149–150, 156–159. (*see also*
  Detoxification program)
  xenoestrogens and, 148–149
Weight Watchers, 189
Wheat, food sensitivities and, 84–86, 131
Wheat protein gluten, 84
Wheezing, 8, 124
White blood cells, 30, 53, 92
White vinegar, 62, 63
Winter months, 30
Withdrawal symptoms, 92, 191
World Health Organization, 86
Wrapping food, 42, 197

Xanax, 238
Xenoestrogens, 41–42, 148–149, 175,
  176, 180
Xylitol, 221

Yeast, 81, 85, 120, 143, 150, 152, 154
Yeast infections, 143
Yerba maté, 194
Yoga, 182
Younger (Thinner) You, The
  (Braverman), 223

Zinc, 68, 71, 167, 188